Social Work and Mental Health

Transforming Social Work Practice – titles in the series

Applied Psychology for Social Work	ISBN: 978 1 84445 071 8
Collaborative Social Work Practice	ISBN: 978 1 84445 014 5
Communication and Interpersonal Skills in Social Work	ISBN: 978 1 84445 019 0
Effective Practice Learning in Social Work	ISBN: 978 1 84445 015 2
Management and Organisations in Social Work	ISBN: 978 1 84445 044 2
Practical Computer Skills for Social Work	ISBN: 978 1 84445 031 2
Social Work and Human Development	ISBN: 978 1 90330 083 1
Social Work and Mental Health (second edition)	ISBN: 978 1 84445 068 8
Social Work in Education and Children's Services	ISBN: 978 1 84445 045 9
Social Work Practice: Assessment, Planning, Intervention and Review	ISBN: 978 1 90330 085 5
Social Work with Children and Families	ISBN: 978 1 84445 018 3
Social Work with Children, Young People and their Families in Scotland	ISBN: 978 1 84445 031 2
Social Work with Drug and Substance Misusers	ISBN: 978 1 84445 058 9
Social Work with Older People	ISBN: 978 1 84445 017 6
Social Work with People with Learning Difficulties	ISBN: 978 1 84445 042 8
Using the Law in Social Work (second edition)	ISBN: 978 1 84445 030 5
Values and Ethics in Social Work	ISBN: 978 1 84445 067 1
What is Social Work? Context and Perspectives (second edition)	ISBN: 978 1 84445 055 1
Youth Justice and Social Work	ISBN: 978 1 84445 066 4

To order, please contact our distributor: BEBC Distribution, Albion Close, Parkstone, Poole, BH12 3LL. Telephone: 0845 230 9000, email: learningmatters@bebc.co.uk. You can also find more information on each of these titles and our other learning resources at www.learningmatters.co.uk.

Social Work and Mental Health

SECOND EDITION

MALCOLM GOLIGHTLEY

Series Editors: Jonathan Parker and Greta Bradley

LearningMatters

First published in 2004 by Learning Matters Ltd.
Reprinted twice in 2005
Second edition published 2006
Reprinted in 2007

© 2006 Malcolm Golightley

British Library Cataloguing in Publication Data
A CIP record for this book is available from the British Library.

ISBN: 978 1 84445 068 8

Cover and text design by Code 5 Design Associates
Project management by Deer Park Productions
Typeset by Pantek Arts Ltd, Kent
Printed and bound in Great Britain by Bell & Bain Ltd, Glasgow

Learning Matters Ltd
33 Southernhay East
Exeter EX1 1NX
Tel: 01392 215560
E-mail: *info@learningmatters.co.uk*
www.learningmatters.co.uk

Contents

Acknowledgements   vi

Introduction   ix

1   Values and ethical mental health social work   1

2   Social work practice and mental health   21

3   The legal and policy context   43

4   Working with vulnerable people: mental health in children and adolescents   71

5   Working with vulnerable people: adults who are short-term service users   95

6   Working with vulnerable people: adults who are long-term service users   115

7   Working across organisational and professional boundaries   133

Glossary   153

References   157

Index   167

Acknowledgements

Thanks are due to the countless people who over the years have maintained my interest in mental health. These have been professionals, volunteers, carers and service users. More specifically thanks are due to Professor Bob Peckitt, consultant psychiatrist at Rampton Hospital whose advice and guidance for Chapter 2 was invaluable; Christopher Curran, a fellow of the University of Lincoln, whose input on the legal chapter was substantial and reflects a number of publications that he and Catherine Grimshaw have produced in Openmind over the last decade; Andy Desiano Plummer and Leonne Griggs for advice and proof reading; and Margaret Lake who graciously allowed me to adapt her stress busting tips. Their advice was invaluable but I take all responsibility for any errors that may be present in the text.

These days life in Higher Education is very full and pressured. There is no spare capacity so writing a book like this not only demands much of one's personal time but of course has an effect on everyone at work. My colleagues at the University of Lincoln deserve many thanks for their support and tolerance.

This book has been a long time in the making but has allowed me to indulge myself in an area which I am passionate about and have been involved in for over 20 years as a practitioner, academic, researcher, and user and carer. I hope the contents do justice to the richness of the experience and to all the things that I have learned from service users and other influential people.

This book is dedicated to my partner Pam, our family, Sharada, Rosie, Sarah, Liam and my grandchildren Kezie Harrison, Maddison Rose and Holly May.

Introduction

This second edition is written primarily for student social workers who are studying for their professional qualification. The second edition contains some of the new policy and legislation that have been introduced since this book first went to print. Whilst it is aimed at first or second year students it will also be useful for the final year and professional practice. The book will appeal to those who work with social workers in the mental health field and to those who are studying related qualifications such as the Certificate in Community Mental Health Care. Experienced and qualified workers should find the content useful for professional updating and to help them understand what students on the new degree are studying.

Requirements for social work education

This book will help students to meet the demands outlined by the Department of Health in the prescribed curriculum and especially in relation to the expressed need that all social workers must understand about mental health and how to work with colleagues from other disciplines.

It will also help meet the Quality Assurance Agency subject benchmarks for social work. These include being able to understand the nature of social work and developing knowledge and understanding about the following:

- social work services and service users;
- values and ethics;
- social work theory; and
- the nature of social work practice.

The National Occupational Standards set for social workers are also covered as the book examines the roles that social workers must play if change and development are to be achieved at an individual, group and service level.

Book structure

Mental health services seem to be in a state of almost continual change. The much-heralded new major legislation has now been shelved leaving the present 20 year old legislation to be amended. Meanwhile new government policies have come into being that will affect both adult services and children and young people services. Although integrated services are high on this agenda it remains my view that social work should be at the heart of these changes and a crucial part of delivering improved services for vulnerable people. This book has in its own modest way a part to play in the transformation of future social work practice.

The beginning of the book has a clear focus upon values and the importance of social workers underpinning their practice with values and principles that demonstrate that they can work with diverse populations, some of whom experience disadvantage and oppression. The examples of work with black and minority ethnic communities and people who are deaf serve to demonstrate the necessity for culturally sensitive practice.

In Chapter 2 the medical model is described in detail as this is the dominant approach to work with service users. However it is not the only approach and the case is put that a more socially oriented approach needs to be understood by social workers as well as the medical approach. This orientation is about more than providing services to support medical interventions: it takes into account a more holistic view of the confusing and contradictory world of mental disorder. To help understand this emphasis is placed on the role that stress has as an intervening variable that increases the vulnerability of people to mental disorder. Such stressful events can include life events or circumstances such as unemployment or relationship breakdown.

The law is never far from mental health social work and Chapter 3 examines the new legal and policy context in which social workers, approved social workers and the putative approved mental health worker will find themselves. The case for and against compulsory admission is made and the process covered. Emphasis is placed on human rights and how they are incorporated into the legislation, and how the various community care initiatives can allow imaginative solutions for helping people return to or remain in the community. The main provisions refer only to the law in England.

Chapter 4 examines work with children and adolescents at a time when *Every Child Matters* has recently come into play and children and young people's services will be altered out of all recognition. Even so, social workers will continue to be among those who will work with a range of mental health disorders that children and young people face. The Child and Adolescent Mental Health Service is a relatively new response and, although slow to get underway, is for the foreseeable future what services will look like. The example of eating disorder is covered in some detail to provide an example of work with adolescents.

Working with service users who are short-term users of mental health services provides the content of Chapter 5. In particular the task facing social workers who are working with people who are at risk of suicide provides the subject matter, with an illustrative example that runs throughout most of the chapter. The importance of understanding the research evidence that frames our work in any area is given emphasis.

Chapter 6 looks at work with service users who have long-term or chronic needs. The illustrative example of a man diagnosed with schizophrenia is used and in particular the concept of early intervention and family work are suggested as ways that effective intervention can be accomplished. Stressful situations can include families that have 'high expressed emotion' and this is used to demonstrate effective work with families. The differences in diagnosis between Afro-Caribbean young men and their white counterparts are explored, and the concept of risk is briefly examined.

The final chapter returns the reader to work with children and the concept of working across professional and organisational boundaries. This covers the importance of child protection and the case of Victoria Climbié. Learning lessons from Inquiries includes learning how to work better together – the Allitt Inquiry raises important issues of which social work professionals should be aware. Children whose parents separate can respond adversely to the stresses that this event can create. Yet others get by and even thrive in later life, and their resilience and ability to bounce back is considered in detail as it provides an important series of pointers as to where intervention could be targeted.

Finally some signposts for the future are aired during the last few pages.

Learning features

As far as a book can be, this has been written to help you to interact with the material as an active participant. The combination of this book, liberal use of the internet and self-reflection should ensure effective learning.

Case studies are used throughout the book to help make real the application of the theory to practice. To add interest some historical notes are provided, especially in Chapter 3.

Throughout this book stress is seen as something that can tip someone from being mentally healthy into having a mental health problem. This can be a single event although often it is a build-up of little things. These need to be dealt with and some chapters provide tips to bust your stress.

Chapter 1
Values and ethical mental health social work

Introduction

The World Heath Organisation describes **mental health** as:

> *a state of well-being in which the individual realizes his or her abilities, can cope with the normal stresses of life, can work productively and fruitfully, and is able to make a contribution to his or her community.*

> *MENTAL ill health includes mental health problems and strain, impaired functioning associated with distress, symptoms, and diagnosable mental health disorders, such as schizophrenia and depression.*

> *The mental condition of people is determined by a multiplicity of factors including biological, individual, family and social, economic and environmental.*
> (European Commission Green Paper, 2005, p.4)

This chapter examines the relationship between values, ethics, contemporary social work and social care practice in the Mental Health Services. Mental health services are at a crucial stage of redevelopment which, by the time it is complete, will produce a service that is appropriate and responsive to service user needs. Values and ethics are at the heart of culturally competent professional practice. This means that social workers will be able to value their own culture and be able to work in a sensitive manner with people from other cultures. To become culturally competent requires empathy, understanding and acceptance of differences. (Walker, 2003; see also culturally sensitive practice in *Engaging and Changing*, Patel, 2003).

Approximately one person in six, at some time in their life, will experience mental health problems that are sufficiently serious for them to seek help from a professional. It is usually the family doctor who is the first port of call and they in turn refer people on to the various agencies whose remit is to provide mental health services. These services include health, social care and social work agencies that are trying to work together to provide a seamless service for the user. Some GP practices have social workers attached to them and this often means that these workers will be doing direct work with service users, working in the community alongside other mental health professionals, or be working in a psychiatric hospital. Social workers also come across mental health problems in addition to the 'presenting problem' that led to referral in the first place.

A strategy for the mental health of the European Union

In January 2005 the World Health Organisation held a conference for European Ministers to start a process of drawing up a framework for comprehensive action and political commitment for mental health. The subsequent Green Paper is an important contribution to setting up a series of actions that may prove to be a significant initiative. The purpose of the Green Paper is to stimulate debate within Europe and to engage a broad range of institutions, health professionals, social care professionals, research communities and service users, in discussions about how best to improve public mental health.

The Green Paper outlines three areas for improvement:

> *Mental ill health affects every fourth citizen and can lead to suicide, a cause of too many deaths.*
>
> *Mental ill health causes significant losses and burdens to the economic, social, educational as well as criminal and justice systems.*
>
> *Stigmatisation, discrimination and non-respect for the human rights and the dignity of mentally ill and disabled people still exist, challenging core European values.*
> (European Commission Green Paper, 2005)

The Paper goes on to describe how mental health is a growing challenge to the EU and to support the WHO view that by 2020 depression will be the highest ranking cause of disease in the developed world (WHO, 2001). Other statistics include the statement that:

> *Currently, in the EU, some 58000 citizens die from suicide every year, more than from the annual deaths from road accidents, homicide or HIV/AIDS.*
> (Green Paper, p.4)

Clearly there are significant inequalities within member states and this reflects the richness of the diverse nature of the EU but nevertheless the Paper proposes that a strategy would be focused upon prevention of mental ill health, the improvement of the quality of life for people with mental health and the development of a mental health information and research system for the EU.

The strategy for England and Wales

The government has set about improving mental health care in general. Key policy documents are *Modernising Mental Health Services* (Department of Health, 1998) and the NHS Plan (Department of Health, 2000). One of the key tasks for the reformed services is to combat the effects of social exclusion and to provide a service that is user-focused. The idea is that through a combination of policy initiatives people will feel that they have a greater sense of belonging to a community and services will form new partnerships between the providers and recipients of services. Thus various initiatives have been put in place to meet the needs of specific populations such as women, people who are deaf, and black and minority ethnic groups.

This more inclusive approach has a focus on community-based services which has been a trend over the last two decades. Prior to this care was provided largely through admission to hospitals, many of which were based on the outskirts of cities and towns. As patients were transferred from hospital to community the danger was that services would become more fragmented. With decentralised structures there is a need to establish general standards against which these communities' services can be judged. The Mental Health National Service Framework (DoH, 1999) is in effect a series of mission statements or targets for services. There are NSFs for mental health, older people, adults and children and young people.

The National Service Framework for adult mental health has seven standards:

- **Standard One** covers mental health promotion and aspects of discrimination and social exclusion that is associated with mental health problems.

- **Standards Two and Three** cover primary care services for people who have mental health problems and include 24-hour crisis services.

- **Standards four and five** highlight what is needed to provide effective services for people with mental health problems. This includes being familiar with the Care Programme Approach and its relation to care management.

- **Standard six** relates to the individuals who care for people with mental health problems, with Social Service Departments being given the lead responsibility in ensuring that all carers' needs are assessed and that they receive their own written care plans.

- **Standard seven** sets out what is needed to achieve a reduction in suicides. This will potentially involve all social workers in a range of settings.

These standards need to be seen alongside the more specific inspection standards such as those of the Commission for Social Care Inspection (CSCI), the successor in April 2004 to the National Care Standards Commission.

Meeting these standards is a challenge to agencies as well as to individual practitioners. As a social worker you may be working with service users and communities as well as other professionals to plan, implement and evaluate mental health services. The emphases on user empowerment, community development and non-discriminatory services are all part of the tool kit that you, as a social worker, will be expected to develop.

Before you can begin to consider yourself an effective mental health social worker you need to understand the values that underpin professional practice and how they are reflected in agency policy and practice and endorsed in governmental policies. You need to understand the part that you will play as a social worker/social care worker in the modernising agenda. It is important that as a developing professional your practice demonstrates commitment to promoting equality.

Two other key policy documents have come into place since the first edition of this book that you will need to familiarise yourself with and these are the Green Paper and the subsequent White Paper known as *Every Child Matters* and for adults the White Paper *Our Health, Our Care, Our Say*: A new direction for community services. Both these documents signal a major change in the way that the Government sees services being provided. They are both accompanied by informative and easy to access websites. As yet many of the implications are still being worked through and you as an emergent professional will be expected to not only understand these changes but also to be a part of the change dynamic.

The importance of policy

Recent policy papers

Present day life in government departments must be a dizzying experience as staff try to produce or perhaps even keep abreast of new initatives. To do so is very important for social workers and as a student you need to develop the habit of reading and critically appraising policy documents and legislation. This is the case even if at first glance such initiatives seem not to be directly related to your area of practice. I have singled out two key papers to help provide the context in which you as a social worker will practice. These are referred to later on in the book but here is a brief summary of the key points.

Our health, our care, our say: a new direction for community services (January, 2006)

This White Paper sets a new direction for the whole health and social care system in respect of adult services. It is founded on the ideas that were consulted on in the Department of Health Green Paper, **Independence, Well-being and Choice (March, 2005)**. The new direction will put service users more than ever at the centre of services which will mean that services will need to be personalised and tailored to ensure that they will fit the service users' needs. Social workers are well placed to work alongside service users to ensure that they become the drivers of service improvement.

The White Paper identifies four main goals:

1. Prevention and early intervention. This will include more support to maintain and even promote mental health and emotional well being.

2. More choice and a louder voice which will aim to provide real choice for service users on a range of services and to provide better information to enable such choices to be made.

3. Inequalities and improving access will focus upon those with ongoing needs in ethnic minorites and young people with disabilities, etc.

4. More support for people with long-term needs so that they can manage their long-term conditions out of hospital and to provide them with a clear plan to help them to promote thier own well being.

Every Child Matters

In 2003 following the death of Victoria Climbié in tragic circumstances, the Goverment published a Green Paper called *Every Child Matters* and once again the tragic circumstances surrounding a child's death and the inadequacies of services led to a major review of provision for children in general. This was aided by an excellent website which you should visit (www.everychildmatters.gov.uk)

Following the consultation, the goverment published *Every Child Matters: the Next Steps*, and passed the Children Act 2004, which set up legislation necessary for developing more effective and accessible services for children, young people and their families.

The commonly held view is that this legislation will transform the provision of services and will change the context in which services are provided irrespective of whether a child or young person has a mental illness, has emotional problems, is socially excluded or in other ways needs their well-being to be enhanced. This new direction offers up the possibility of more integrated services which are fit for purpose.

The five outcomes set out by ECM are:

- Being healthy
- Staying safe

- Enjoying and achieving
- Making a positive contribution
- Social and economic well-being.

The importance of values

Social work is fundamentally a moral activity. Social workers often refer to values, indeed Clark (2000) suggests that values are the staple diet of social workers although the word is used indiscriminately when principles or ethics would be more accurate. Clark suggest that there are four core values:

1. The worth and uniqueness of each individual.

2. The entitlement to justice.

3. The essentiality of community.

4. The claim to freedom.

These values are given statutory force through the National Health Service and Community Care Act (DoH, 1990) and various practice guidance notes including Valuing People (DoH, 2001) that stress not only the importance of these values but require services and practitioners to uphold them.

Values, knowledge and skills are interconnected in everyday practice even though this is not always apparent. Figure 1 shows how these are connected to each other.

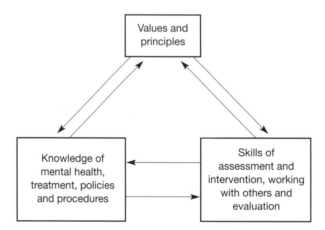

Figure 1.1 *Values, knowledge and skills: the foundations of good practice*

All social care workers will be required in the future to register with the General Social Care Council, starting in April 2005 with social workers. Once this process is complete it will allow external confirmation that a member of staff is registered and suitably qualified. This process regulates who can and who cannot enter the profession and is considered necessary in order to drive up the standards of social work and social care practice (Banks, 2000).

The need for a Code of Professional Practice becomes apparent when you begin to learn about the role that social workers have alongside other professionals who deliver mental health services. At times people with mental health problems can be in such a vulnerable state that they may even require admission to hospital against their wishes. They need to be assured that nationally agreed standards of service delivery are being adhered to and that the service provider can be held accountable when services fall short. Different professions have their own codes of practice and conduct which have three common themes:

- the avoidance of possible harm to services users;
- the promotion of possible good to service users;
- the protection of the profession and the resolution of conflicts.

How are you going to be guided by values and ethics?

The Code sets out the responsibilities for both employers and employees as follows.

Social care workers must:

- Protect the rights and promote the interests of service users and carers.
- Strive to establish and maintain the trust and confidence of service users and carers.
- Promote the independence of service users while protecting them as far as possible from danger and harm.
- Respect the rights of service users whilst seeking to ensure that their behaviour does not harm themselves or other people.
- Uphold public trust and confidence in social care services.
- Be accountable for the quality of their work and take responsibility for maintaining and improving their knowledge and skills.

ACTIVITY *1.1*

Look at your Code of Practice which sets out the kind of professional conduct and practice that is required (GSCC, 2002). You should have a copy of this Code but if not you can print it off the GSCC website or obtain a hard copy from them: General Social Care Council, Goldings House, 2 Hay's Lane, London SE1 2BH. Tel: 020 7397 5100. Email: info@gscc.org.uk www.gscc.org.uk

Make sure that you are aware of the contents of the Code.

Look at the above Code. Taking all the aspects reorder them to fit into the framework proposed earlier:

- *ones that avoid possible harm to service users;*
- *ones that promote possible good to service users;*
- *ones that protect the profession and resolve conflicts.*

Values in action

Implicit in the Code of Professional Social Work Practice is the importance of recognising and respecting diversity. This is more than valuing people irrespective of their race, colour or ability. It also involves valuing and respecting that people think and behave differently. People of all ethnic backgrounds and countries experience mental disorder and the service user population is made up of people just like you and me.

Conventionally and stereotypically medical practice has remained the dominant partner through its claim to be a series of technical activities. Advances in medication have reinforced the idea that an individual's mental disorder can be managed and that the key process is diagnosis followed by treatment monitoring and evaluation. In this process the danger is that the treated are subservient to those in charge of treatment.

Social workers need to work with medical and health colleagues to provide an effective service but they also need to be at the forefront of processes that empower service users. Implicit in this approach are some ordinary but powerful principles.

The first is that in order to empower someone we need to work with them rather than do things to them. Empowerment means partnership, openness and honesty.

The second principle is that the service user has an explanation of their disorder. That needs understanding and to achieve this we need to find ways of active listening that respect the user and enable us to do our job. This may mean having to use imaginative ways of communicating. It might mean trying to use a common language, which could be sign language. It should mean engaging in clear, uncomplicated language that everyone can understand.

The third principle is that service users value being able to engage with professionals on a personal level. This could mean that social workers should learn to use 'limited' self-disclosure to help build up professional relationships that are also person-to-person, not expert to amateur (Blackburn and Golightley, 2004). Being able to walk in the other person's shoes is an important part of an empowering approach.

The fourth principle is that the service user is the expert in their own mental health problem. They may not know the answers but they certainly experience the effect or symptoms. They alone have experienced the disintegration of 'normality' as they know it and their explanation should be put alongside the professional view and the two views evaluated against each other. If your world is upside down or inside out it cannot be understood by people who only see things one way up or right side out. If a service user is hearing voices the social worker must not dismiss these but try to understand when they arrive, what they feel like and how best they can be managed. This is not to collude with delusional behaviour as this could be unhelpful and possibly run the risk of missing dangerous behaviour.

By working with service users to value their experiences, and by seeing the problem through their eyes, the prospect is opened up to work in a manner that is holistic and empowering.

Ethical dilemmas

Health and social care workers work with dilemmas on a daily basis. There are usually two components that help us to think about ethical dilemmas. First there may be competing views about what should be done. How would you respond to a service user when they want to stop taking their medicine? This is an ethical dilemma and people would argue strongly for one position or the other. This contrasts with a view that medicine should be given with or without service user consent, if it were necessary to prevent death or serious harm occurring. In this instance this is not an ethical issue as there is widespread agreement. (Even so some people claim this should not happen, usually on religious grounds.)

The second characteristic is that it must have a distinct moral component to it, such as the avoidance of lying, the primacy of life, self-determination and confidentiality. These are sometimes referred to as 'normative principles'.

Resolving ethical dilemmas takes more than just referring to these normative principles or the various codes of conduct. It requires professional judgments after weighing up one principle against another. The following activity will help you to think further about the ethical dilemmas.

ACTIVITY **1.2**

Sanjay is a long-term service user who has recurring bouts of depression, which are serious enough to warrant his treatment with anti-depressants. In the past when his mood has been very low he has talked about 'ending it all'. As his social worker you visit regularly and he tells you in confidence that he has stopped his medication and is going to experiment with herbal medicine which is more usual in his culture. He has asked your opinion about this action and told you to keep this conversation confidential. Should you respect his wishes? Jot down what your response would be and what the issues are. Now compare with the following paragraphs.

If anyone wants to stop taking medication then this is their right under common law. In certain circumstances, and providing that they are detained under the Mental Health Act 1983, they can be made to have treatment against their wishes. Sanjay can stop his medication although whether this is a good thing is open to debate.

Arguments against keeping confidences or keeping matters confidential derive from different sources. First there is a principle of paternalism usually derived from the possession of 'expert' knowledge. Put crudely the professional knows best. Second there is a principle of autonomy where the person has freedom over his or her own body, which is essentially a moral principle. Individuals are experts in their own mental health condition and as such they know best. Resolution of this requires you to balance the strength of one principle against the other. In practice you would probably seek to encourage Sanjay to sit with the others involved in his treatment and to talk through his and your concerns and try to get to a position where his shift to herbal remedies is informed by evidence, monitored and reviewed.

You would need to take into account the extent to which the service user has the capacity to be able to make such a decision, the quality of the information on which this is based, if there was any coercion on the service user when making this decision and any legal issues that could change the nature of the discussion.

One way that service users can be helped to make good quality decisions is through patient advocacy services. By using advocates who are independent of the mental health team, but who have specific knowledge of mental health and mental health services, the quality of service user decisions can be enhanced.

Ethnicity and mental health

The discrimination that is experienced by people with mental health problems can be intensified if that person happens to be from a black and minority ethnic community. A service user talks about her experience of using mental health services as a black person:

> *Coming to mental health services was like the last straw ... you come to services disempowered already, they strip you of your dignity ... you become the dregs of society.* (Keating and Robertson, 2002, p.18)

This is a commonly held experience of black service users. When put together with the perception that when black people are seen as difficult they are likely to be over medicated there is little wonder that this has become a priority area.

Discrimination has been a source of concern to many practitioners over the years. Evidence has suggested that on the one hand the UK's black and minority ethnic population are over-represented in secondary care (hospital admissions etc) and on the other hand under-represented in primary care that specifically addresses the needs of black and minority ethnic communities. Of particular concern has been the over-representation of Caribbean and black African people who have been detained against their will and who are being treated in Medium Secure Hospitals (MSUs). Evidence collected by the Mental Health Act Commission shows that 30% of the population resident in MSUs were from predominantly black African or Caribbean ethnic groups, which is well over the proportion that might be expected when compared with the population at large.

Fundamental to developing better social work practice is having better quality of information and using it more intelligently than is evident at present. A starting point is for you to become familiar with population data and information about ethnic minorities.

ACTIVITY **1.3**

The proportion of black and minority ethnic groups in the UK rose from 6% to 9% over the period 1991–2001. The Afro-Caribbean population in England and Wales is about 2%. This does vary considerably depending on where you live and work. Commonly members of the public at large over-estimate the numbers of black and minority ethnic populations. Think about why this is, what influences this perception and what some of the implications of this might be. Write down why you think some ethnic groups are thought to be larger than they actually, are, what influences this perception and some of the implications of this.

You probably came up with the idea that the media plays a big role here with some of the less sophisticated newspapers in particular promoting the idea that we are being overpopulated with asylum seekers, drug users and the like. Mental health is not the only area where we see statistics that ought to concern us: the *Sunday Times* (Dec 14, 2003) reported, 'twice as many black people are in prison as at university'. They report that the Race Relations watchdog has concluded that while 10,000 Afro-Caribbeans are in jails – a much higher percentage than to be expected – the numbers at university are only about 5,000.

Providing mental health services that are, and need to be seen to be, responsive to the needs of individuals requires that they should reflect the rich diversity that makes up our society. However in the late 1980s it was becoming apparent that although moves were being made to promote patient-centred services this did nothing to address the specific needs of the black and minority ethnic communities.

Although these views were commonly held throughout health and social care, social work was one of the few professions that placed special emphasis on training in anti-racist and anti-discriminatory practice. At the policy level, the government's Modernisation Plan and the Mental Health National Service Framework (1999) sets out in Standard One the need to combat discrimination against individuals and groups with mental health problems and promote their social inclusion. This has built on the legal foundation laid down in the Human Rights Act 1998 and is given extra strength by the introduction of the Race Relations (Amendment) Act 2000.

More recently the Department of Health has set out an impressive and ambitious change agenda called *Delivering Race Equality: A Framework for Action* (October 2003). Although this is a consultation document, and may be amended, it is likely that the general approach and principles will remain.

What does this mean for mental health social work practice?

James Nazroo (1999) suggests that different rates of diagnosis of mental illness between black and minority ethnic people represents one of the most controversial issues that present day services face. In practical terms you need to examine the reasons why minority groups such as Afro-Caribbean men are six times more likely to be compulsorily detained than white people, why Asian women are more likely to be depressed than their white counterparts and why minority ethnic groups are less likely to seek early help from primary care.

Mental health is a significant area of social work practice, which will bring you face to face with people who may be vulnerable and confused. As a social worker you need to work together with other professionals in a way that is person-centred and upholds human rights. This is far from straightforward, with tension and conflict possible at virtually every stage of your work. Such tension can exist between for example:

• the wishes of the service user and their families;

• the need to protect the public and the need to promote service user independence;

• and, as you saw earlier, the right to refuse treatment and the need to have treatment.

In trying to work with these tensions you will often find yourself playing a crucial role in any decision-making context.

Anti-oppressive practice

Social work has a history of attempts to practise in ways that are anti-oppressive. One of the key figures in the literature is Dominelli whose book *Anti-Racist Social Work* (1988) not only provides well argued discussion about these issues but also gives strategies for the implementation of anti-racist social work. These ideas, although nearly two decades old, still have relevance for you as a practitioner as mental health care is the only aspect of care provision and treatment that, if refused, can result in that person's compulsory admission to hospital through a legally authorised pathway. Social workers, after suitable post-qualifying training, can be a major part of such procedures and can also be involved in other aspects such as providing advocacy, reports for tribunals, arranging diversion into community resources, etc.

ACTIVITY **1.4**

Think of a situation where, in practical terms, you will have to take culture into account when working with someone from a black and minority ethnic background.

There will be lots of examples that you could give and one is when compiling a Social Circumstances Report for a Mental Health Review Tribunal. Tribunals take place when someone has been detained in a psychiatric facility and wishes to appeal against this detention. The Tribunals consider various reports including ones compiled by social workers. These are formal reports that are presented to the Tribunal and they are a part of the mechanism by which compulsorily detained patients can be discharged from hospital. These reports provide the Tribunal with the cultural background of the service user and describe past patterns of behaviour that can help to determine the likely success of aftercare, together with other salient details such as accommodation and employment opportunities.

The Mental Health Act Code of Practice sets out as a guiding principle that all people should be respected for their:

> *... diverse backgrounds as individuals and be assured that account will be taken of their age, gender, sexual orientation, social, ethnic, cultural and religious background, but that general assumptions will not be made on the basis of any one of these characteristics.*
> (DoH, 1999, p.3)

This latter point is especially relevant as there is a risk of assuming cultural stereotypes, which can not only cause offence but can be widely misleading. In any event understanding someone's culture is only a first step towards anti-oppressive practice.

Are black and minority ethnic people the only community who get poorer services than the majority population? The answer is a qualified no! Other groups include older people, children and adolescents, women and people who are deaf. All these groups are covered in this book but working with mental health users who are deaf raises some interesting parallels with working with black and minority ethnic users as well as some challenges for you to face in your practice.

Deaf people and mental health

CASE STUDY

There are limited specialist services available for deaf people who have severe mental illness. This was highlighted by the Independent Inquiry into the care and treatment of Daniel Joseph (Mischoh, 2000), which was commissioned by some of the London Health Authorities. Daniel was profoundly deaf and was admitted to hospital from the courts having been made subject to a hospital order with restrictions after pleading guilty to manslaughter with diminished responsibility. Concern over his treatment resulted in the present government consulting about services across the spectrum for service users who are deaf.

People who are deaf, like black and minority ethnic people, report that mental health services are difficult to access and often do not cater for their specific needs. To raise our awareness of the specific needs of minority communities the Department of Health consultation paper *A Sign of the Times: Modernising mental health services for people who are deaf* (DoH, 2002) is worth consulting. Developing awareness of specific communities is an important, but only a first, step towards developing appropriate and responsive services.

The Royal National Institute for Deaf People estimates that there are eight million people who suffer from hearing loss, often associated with aging, and that there are about 50,000 people for whom British Sign Language is their first and preferred language (RNID, 2003).

Members of the deaf community experience mental health problems just like people from any other community. However because of the difference in language and culture between those who are assessing deaf service users and the service users themselves, misdiagnosis can result and as a consequence deaf people can receive services and treatment that are inappropriate. Good practice needs to take into consideration the requirements of the Disability Discrimination Act (DoH,1999) which makes it clear that mental health services have to take reasonable steps to facilitate the uptake of services by people who are deaf and who have mental health problems (sometimes referred to as people with dual diagnosis). This includes the use of an interpreter at the various stages of assessment and provision of services.

Culture is a central feature of a person's identity and that at the very least must be taken into consideration when working with service users from black and minority ethnic communities or when working with service users who are deaf.

Does the relative social exclusion that deaf people experience contribute to their mental health problems? This is reported as being a factor in the relationship between the psychological health of deaf people and their subsequent call upon mental health services. In other words being deaf can increase your vulnerability to mental health problems (Ridgeway, 1997). In Chapter 2 explanations are given of the cause and manifestation of mental health problems and in particular the role that stress plays in mental health.

Until recently mental health services seemed to be based around the assumptions that users were all from a hearing population that is predominantly white British. Both of these assumptions are well off the mark and need to be challenged and changed. To meet the NSF Standard One services need to be provided that are sensitised to the needs of different people. In reality the respect for the person's cultural identity is the predominant value that ought to underpin your practice.

CASE STUDY

Shaz is a deaf person who lives alone and, at the age of 32, has very few connections with the deaf community. She is a fluent user of British Sign Language but since her remand to prison on theft charges her health has suffered. Over the last ten years or so she has been treated for depression and has taken anti-depressants. The stress of being in prison has caused her more distress to the extent that she would like to see a social worker. However the prison service does not have a person who can sign and therefore they must seek outside specialist support. By chance the local community mental health team has a member of staff who can sign and she accompanies the social worker to the prison and carries out an assessment with the prison doctor.

This example shows how services can respond in an ideal way. However having a person who can effectively communicate in the same language as the service user is often a matter of luck and there is a need for more services of this nature. A deaf person who communicates through sign language is likely to find that being in an environment where fluent signers are is more conducive to their recovery than being in a hearing world. Of course once the specialist worker leaves the prison Shaz is left still having to cope with the traumas of prison, which is essentially a hearing world. This still leaves you having to explore with Shaz and the interpreter what specific needs she might have in respect to her deafness.

Learning disability and mental health

People who have a learning disability can experience a range of mental health problems just like the rest of us. However the presence of learning disability may prevent professionals and carers recognising the symptoms of mental health problems such as depression. It is important for carers and professionals to look beyond stereotypes and seek explanations for behaviour that has typically changed. Finding out what is wrong will call for quality communication and observation skills and working in a partnership with carers and service users. There are some informative guides published by the Royal College of Psychiatrists and the likes of MENCAP most of which you can download from their websites.

There are few research and evaluation studies in the field of learning disability and mental health – dual diagnosis is the technical term often used. This tends to maintain this important area as low priority yet Government policy expounded in the White Paper Valuing People urges people with learning difficulties to use mainstream NHS services. This of course includes mental health services. (Valuing People, March 2001)

The coexistence of mental health problems alongside learning disability may be one of the explanations of the existence of challenging behaviour. Such behaviour may not be a characteristic of learning disability but may be as a result of mental health problems. This is a theme that Moss picks up in his article in the *British Journal of Psychiatry*, which showed that there was 'some evidence for a statistical association between challenging behaviour and psychiatric disorder' (Moss, p.454). They concluded that depression was four times more prevalent in people with learning disability who exhibited challenging behaviour than for people with learning disability itself. This finding, although needing to be treated with some caution, is important as depression is so often overlooked in people with learning disability.

Working with service users who have this form of dual diagnosis often will mean mobilising community resources to provide support and connection with others in the community. This idea of connectedness is described by Peter Gilbert: 'Mental distress and mental illness is so often about a disconnection, false connections or an over concentration on one aspect of our lives'. (page 22). Like any other service user you as a social worker will want to access the whole person and how they draw support or otherwise from their families, carers and the community. Facilitating better connections within the community may be the most appropriate intervention that you can make.

Culturally competent practice: transforming social work

Cultural competence is a bringing together of some of the big ideas covered in this chapter. It is a combination of:

- awareness;

- knowledge of anti-oppressive practice;

- values based practice;

- interpersonal skills that will provide you with the basic building blocks of a practice that is appropriate; and

- sensitivity to working with service users who may not always be from your own culture.

A culturally competent service can be defined as one that is perceived by minority ethnic users

---

CASE STUDY

Christopher Clunis – inadequate care and treatment?

Christopher Clunis is a young Afro-Caribbean man who had a history of severe mental illness. He had been diagnosed as having paranoid schizophrenia when he lived in Jamaica. In December 1992 he attacked and killed Jonathon Zito who was completely unknown to him.

The subsequent inquiry has been widely reported and some of the findings reveal the perils of professional practice that is not culturally relevant.

CASE STUDY *continued*

The inquiry team concluded that:

The added factor of his blackness may have contributed to the diffident manner in which some professionals treated him and it may have caused them to defer against his best interests, to his own expressed wishes.
(Ritchie et al., 1994, p.4)

and

Young black males should not be type-cast as suffering from schizophrenia unless the clinical indications warrant it and clinicians and others who care for black mentally ill people should not be too ready to ascribe odd behaviour to the abuse of drugs.
(Ritchie et al., 1994, p.129)

---

as being appropriate to their cultural and religious beliefs and responsive to their needs.

This case study shows the extent to which stereotypical views can permeate professional practice and it highlights the dangers of seeing people only by the colour of their skin. Looking beyond this in a critical manner is the hallmark of good practice. At this point it is appropriate to examine the ways in which our practice can be transformed.

It should be clear that services need to become more relevant to the needs of black and minority ethnic groups and other minority groups such as people who are deaf. Service users frequently point out that the services that they are receiving show little understanding of their culture. But changing this is not a simple matter. You also need to recognise that this is a sensitive issue influenced by your own ethnicity and skin colour. Social workers who are skilled in anti-oppressive practice and using a values based practice approach are clearly further on than those who are not, but there is no room for complacency as many of the explanations of service variability show that racism permeates organisations.

It is questionable whether we can be competent in cultures that are not our own and in any case the range of diverse cultures in the UK makes competence in all cultures an unrealistic proposition. An alternative to understanding different cultures is to recruit more social workers and other professionals from these minority communities to ensure cultural congruence or, in other words, proportionate representation of professionals from all groups. However this can only be a limited strategy, for although positive action strategies when recruiting staff and adopting equal opportunities interview methods are vitally important, they are in themselves insufficient.

But what if you are a black social worker working with white service users or the other way around? What kind of approach can you adopt? To what extent do your stereotypes distort your assessment and decision-making processes? The National Institute for Mental Health England (NIMHE) has recommended that all staff working in this area receive compulsory training in cultural awareness to help eradicate racism and discrimination. Although there are many such courses around quite a few of these promote awareness rather than competency. Awareness is just one stage in developing culturally competent practice.

Components of culturally competent practice

The idea of being able to work with a diverse range of cultures is not entirely new but has gained momentum and acceptance of late. Walker (2003) uses the idea of cultural competence building on the work of Kim (1995), while Patel et al. in *Engaging and Changing* (2003) refer to practice as being 'culturally sensitive', whereas Fulford (in MHAC 10th Biennial 2001–2003) describes 'value based practice'. Some of the common themes are blended together into five components of culturally competent practice and each of these is explored below.

Capacity for your own cultural awareness
This should start with an honest understanding of your own culture and the impact that this has on your professional practice. You need to be aware of your own attitudes, values and beliefs before you can be aware of the attitudes and beliefs of others.

Capacity for awareness of other cultures
It is a widely held view that self-awareness is one of the core components of a practice that is culturally competent (O'Hagan, 2001; Poole, 1998, etc.) but after that it is necessary for you to develop your own capacity for understanding the other cultures and putting this understanding into practice. This requires you to make a realistic assessment of your knowledge and understanding of working with people and of their cultures.

Understanding of diversity and difference
Community engagement is currently being promoted as the main way that professionals can increase their understanding of specific needs of communities. Social workers should respect diversity and build upon people's strengths and the collective strengths of the communities. Effective work with and across cultures requires that you understand and value difference both at the individual and at the community level. This also means recognising and accepting your own personal and professional limitations.

Transferring skills from one service user culture to another
At the heart of much of professional practice is the idea that skills that are learned from work with one type of problem can be transferred to another. This means that the skills that you have in assessing white people who have depression can also be used when working with Asian people who have depression. But as we have seen earlier effective assessment requires you to understand the context in which the person is living. However social work skills such as empowering practice are key components of this transforming practice.

Being able to recognise the impact of structural racism and discrimination
Section 11 of the Health and Social Care Act 2001 places a duty on local health services to consult with services users and the public in the planning and development of services and this is an important step in the development of better and more appropriate services. Services are required to work *with* vulnerable groups and individuals at risk and to tackle social exclusion. This means that all providers of mental health services, including GPs and primary care workers, will be involved in some way or other in helping to deliver a service that is culturally appropriate and responsive to all groups in society.

Is it possible to achieve cultural competence?

The Government has established a five-year action plan called Delivering Race Equality in Mental Health Care, which is the main driver behind the attempt to achieve a culturally more responsive and capable workforce. As you can see from the list set out earlier this is a difficult task and not everyone thinks this will be achieved.

An interesting article in the *Guardian* should give cause for some healthy scepticism, a small extract of which follows:

> *Joanna Bennett, who leads research on workforce development at the Sainsbury Centre for Mental Health, has completed a review of race-related training and thinks that the picture is of 'a lot of fragmentation, different approaches and different models'. She says: 'There is no agreed definition of cultural competence and no evidence that it works in producing better services for black and minority ethnic users. We should be looking at structural processes and power relationships in the way services are delivered.'*

Bennett, a psychiatric nurse and former lecturer in mental health at Middlesex University, is the sister of David Bennett who died while in the care of mental health services. In evidence to the inquiry into his death, she warned against services focusing on 'cultural matching' in favour of staff spending more time talking to patients and thier families. Taking time to respect an individual, and ask what was troubling him and what he needed, was likely to be more effective than 'talking about culture, ethnicity and cultural competence' (*Guardian* Wednesday, 2006 April 12)

The significance of the above is that the inquiry into the death of Bennett, who had schizophrenia and who died during a restraint procedure at a medium secure unit, was that training for cultural competence was one of their high priority training recommendations. This followed the discovery during the inquiry that very little attempt had been made to understand let alone relate to the racial and cultural needs of David Bennett.

Achieving cultural competence may well require more than individuals alone can achieve although as Joanna Bennett points out getting the basis right will go a long way towards providing a more user focused service.

Promoting your own mental health

As you go through your course you are likely to be living a multitude of roles and having to meet numerous deadlines and expectations. These could include working to supplement your bursary or grant; balancing family life with college demands; worry about passing assignments and much more. Stress plays a big part in our own mental health and concern has risen in recent years over the increase in reported mental health problems for students in colleges and universities. In my experience social work students are no different from the majority of students studying on a variety of courses.

Students come to study at UK universities from all over the world and as a consequence the student community is as diverse as if not more so than the community at large. While many students can draw upon a range of personal resources, some are a long way from the support systems that have previously nurtured them. There are cultural differences which also may mean that they are unwilling to talk about personal issues with comparative strangers. It could also be that those who could offer help and may be concerned do not recognise the signs or mistakenly interpret these signs as cultural differences.

It might be that you recognise some of these elements in yourself and that you are reluctant to seek help, partly because of the possible impact on your studies. If this is getting to be a serious problem you should seek help as social work is a stressful career and you need early on to develop strategies that will enhance your own mental health for dealing with such stresses.

It is unlawful for universities to treat students with mental health problems that are substantial, adverse and long-term (more than 12 months) less favourably by excluding them temporarily or permanently if the reason is their mental health. Consequently a university should not exclude a student if their disruptive behaviour is primarily caused by mental health that falls into the realm of the Disability Discrimination Act 1995 (amended by the Special Educational Needs and Disability Act 2001).

Stress busting tip
The boxes technique

Think of a problem that you are currently dealing with (or have been recently) that has been causing you some concern, and how your mind goes over and over the problem. If that happens to you it can become stressful and unproductive. It can also prevent you from getting on with other things as your mind is focused on seemingly difficult problems. In time if this continues it can produce stress and perhaps sleepless nights. This is one technique for controlling and organising these problems that has been tried and tested by many students over the years.

1. Close your eyes and imagine that your mind is divided into a series of boxes and that each box has a lid.

2. Take each problem and place it into its own box.

3. Firmly place a lid on each box.

4. You now have your problems under control.

5. Only allow yourself to remove one lid at a time.

6. You can now focus all your attention on your released problem.

7. You may feel some of the lids on the other boxes starting to rise, if so be firm and replace them telling yourself that you will focus upon them at a later time. Persistent lid risers need a heavy weight to be placed upon them.

8. This technique really does work better with practice and students report that it is a good stress buster.

RESEARCH SUMMARY

The Mental Health Foundation commissioned research to overview current research and mental health initiatives related to student mental health. Among the findings was that clinical depression was reported in 12% of male students and 15% of females. This is an increase over the last time such estimates were made in 1987.

Student counsellors also reported an increase in the proportion of students with severe mental health problems or disorder. At the extreme end suicide among students has risen from 2.4 per 100,000 to 9.7. This is over the ten-year period 1983–1993/4.

(Fox, P. et al. in mentalhealth.org.uk/page.cfm?pagecode=PBUP0211)

C H A P T E R   S U M M A R Y

We have seen the impact that values and ethics have on mental health social work. These values are set down by the professional bodies and in the case of social work by the General Social Care Council.

Transforming social work in the twenty-first century requires workers to be able to recognise their own prejudices and biases and to move beyond these to develop a practice that is culturally competent, demonstrated by the worker's awareness of the service user's culture, including religion and traits. It also means looking after your own mental health and recognising that we all are susceptible to various mental health problems.

Transforming practice means also engaging in more than the rhetoric of anti-oppressive practice and value-based practice. It means demonstrating that these major ideas have influenced everyday mental health work. This means seeing the person not just as the mental health problem that they exhibit and not being influenced by stereotypes. Listening to what users have to say about their experiences is an important part of this process.

FURTHER READING

Department of Health (October 2003) *'Delivering Race Equality: A framework for action consultation document'*. London: DoH. A consultation document that sets out the 9 building blocks of improved practice for mental health services.

The Mental Health Act Code of Practice (DoH, 1999) gives specific practice guidelines when working with service users who are detained in psychiatric hospitals or units. It covers a range of activities including medication, other forms of treatment, control and restraint and what constitutes an emergency. This is essential reading for those who intend to practise in a mental health setting. NHS Trusts are advised to ensure that all staff undertake training in the meaning of the Code.

WEBSITES

The Internet Encyclopaedia of Philosophy has several pages concerned with the field of ethics and is a good place to visit for more information about 'normative principles in applied ethics'. www.utm.edu/research/iep/e/ethics.htm

Fox, P. et al. in mentalhealth.org.uk/page.cfm?pagecode=PBUP0211

RNID: fact sheet Introducing British Sign Language can be download free from www.ucl.ac.uk/library

Chapter 2
Social work practice and mental health

This chapter will help you to begin to meet the following National Occupational Standards:

Key Role 1: Prepare for and work with individuals, families, carers, groups and communities to assess their needs and circumstances
- Assess needs and options to recommend a course of action.

Key Role 2: Plan, carry out, review and evaluate social work practice, with individuals, families, carers, groups and communities and other professionals
- Interact with individuals, families, carers, groups and communities to achieve change and development and to improve life opportunities.
- Address behaviour which presents a risk to individuals, families, carers, groups and communities.

Key Role 6: Demonstrate professional competence in social work practice
- Research, analyse, evaluate and use current knowledge of best social work practice.
- Work within agreed standards of social work practice and ensure own professional development.

It will also introduce you to the following academic standards as set out in the social work subject benchmark statement, which includes:

2.2.2 Defining principles

There are competing views in society at large about the nature of social work and its place and purpose. Social work practice and education inevitably reflect these differing perspectives on the role of social work in relation to social justice, social care and social order.

3.1.1 Social work services and service users
- The nature and validity of different definitions of, and explanations for, the characteristics and circumstances of service users and the services required by them.

3.1.4 Social work theory
- Research-based concepts and critical explanations from social work theory and other disciplines that contribute to the knowledge base of social work, including their distinctive epistemological status and application to practice.
- The relevance of sociological perspectives to understanding societal and structural influences on human behaviour at individual, group and community levels.
- The relevance of psychological and physiological perspectives to understanding individual and social development and functioning.

The subject skills highlighted to demonstrate this knowledge in practice include:
- Assessing human situations, taking into account a variety of factors.
- Assessing the merits of contrasting theories.

Introduction

The greatest happiness of the greatest number is the foundation of morals and legislation.
Jeremy Bentham. (1832)

This chapter introduces you to what is meant by mental illness and mental health. The dominant model of mental illness is medical, which is explored here. The importance of understanding not only what various diagnoses mean but also the implications of adopting the medical model is assessed. A contrasting perspective that incorporates social differences including gender, ethnicity, and age is also explored. Overlaid onto these differences are the social structural explanations that revolve around social exclusion and isolation, which will build on the foundations laid in Chapter 1.

This is not a medical text and you should use this text to guide your study rather than as a sole resource.

What is meant by mental illness and mental health?

The first point that needs to be made is that there are different terms currently used to describe the same thing. For example you will hear terms such as mental distress, mental illness, mental disorder, mental health problems, mental health challenges, all used by students and professionals.

In this book the following terms are used.

Mental disorder is a broad term that covers any significant departure from a state of 'normal' health and includes diseases and illness. These include severe forms like schizophrenia and manic depression. Mental disorder implies that a state of 'normality' once existed and therefore offers the chance to work with the person to restore them to that state, and is usually a temporary condition.

Mental health is a difficult term to be categorical about as it is far more than the absence of illness. I suggest that it is about achieving your potential as a human being. People can have mental health problems, which are 'problems of everyday life' which just have to be got on with.

Learning disability (formerly known as mental handicap and before that as mental deficiency). With learning disability the individual's rate of progress is slower than for most and treatment is not about a cure, as this is a long-term, permanent, condition, but about providing an environment in which the individual can achieve their potential.

RESEARCH STATISTICS

In 2000 the Office for National Statistics (ONS) carried out a survey of psychiatric morbidity of people aged 16 to 74 years living in private households in Great Britain, and it found that about one in six adults aged between 16 and 74 living in private households had a neurotic disorder, such as depression, anxiety or a phobia.

Lifetime experience of stressful life events: by type of event and gender, 2000: Social Trends 32

There are numerous perspectives about mental health and you need to get a good understanding of the various 'models' that are in current use. This means that you can evaluate one against the other and more importantly begin to put your practice in an appropriate framework. To help your understanding the **social model** and the **medical model** are described as two key perspectives that inform work with service users who have mental disorder.

First we should consider from where the general public gets information about mental disorder: by and large, through the media. The lay perspective, as it might be called, is important and few studies have examined how people conceptualise mental health. One of the few studies in this area showed that mental illness and mental health are seen by the public as being part of the same continuum and have negative connotations.

ACTIVITY **2.1**

Messages in the media

Think about the media coverage of mental illness and jot down the memorable words. Can you remember the last time that you read an article that was using positive adjectives or celebrating the success of people with mental health problems? What terms are used to portray mental health? Does this portrayal vary from media source to media source, from tabloid to serious newspapers?

You may well have written down terms like 'nutter' or 'looney' which are in common use and have negative connotations. These are some of the ways that behaviours can become associated with certain labels and consequently become self-fulfilling prophecies. What are your views about this? Is calling someone a 'nutter' just a piece of harmless fun or does it bring with it unwanted labels?

Words that are used by the media and in particular the tabloid press are often associated with violence and risk. Even though the risk of a stranger who is mentally ill killing you is very small, some of the press coverage suggests that it is a common occurrence.

Finally you might find it interesting to look at coverage in the press over the next few weeks and compare different newspapers and, if you have the time, think about how you would rewrite the headline or sub-heads.

Explaining mental health

It is easy to see that there are two perspectives about what causes mental health:

- that held by the medical practitioners which is essentially a biomedical or disease model;
- and that held by professionals like social workers which looks at social causation and/or labelling as explanations.

This separation into one or the other model is probably only useful in an academic or research sense as the medical perspective dominates and other perspectives need to at least take this perspective on board. This is now explored.

The medical model

This is a medical perspective that is adopted by doctors and psychiatrists and is sometimes called the 'disease model'. The acceptance of this model gives credence to the claim that organic or biomedical causes will eventually be found for all forms of mental disorder. Although the psychiatric model dominates discourse about mental disorder, this is as much by accident as it is by virtue of its conceptual strength. Andrew Scull, in his book *Museums of Madness* (1979), describes how a transformation occurred from people being seen as eccentrics, village fools or possessed by the demon when, around 150 years ago, the state took control and the medical profession was employed to treat and manage mental disorder.

In contemporary practice social workers work alongside other health professionals including psychiatrists to deliver mental health services. At some point you will be involved in an assessment of what the service users' needs are, which may necessitate a diagnosis.

Assessment

As a social worker you are most likely to be involved in this early stage of assessment and treatment of mental disorder. Campbell (1999) suggests that social workers can only become competent when, as a practitioner, they are able to synthesise interpersonal skills with theories and ideas about the causes of mental disorder. This is the case for all settings and aspects of the work. You may also be involved later in your career as an Approved Social Worker or similar with specific responsibilities under the legislation to assess a service user for whom compulsory admission to hospital may be the last resort. This is covered in the chapter on legal issues. An in-depth assessment would need to include some or all of the following:

- previous history of mental health problems or difficulties;
- service user self-assessment of their difficulties;
- cultural and religious aspects;
- employment status;
- relationship strengths and weaknesses;
- substance use or misuse including drug and alcohol use.

The importance of this approach is to identify what would be considered to be the most effective way of proceeding with the service user. The aim is to work in a manner that the service user would describe as culturally sensitive and which focuses upon the service user's strengths rather than deficits. Service users who have experienced mental health problems may have also experienced what works for them and your task may be one of mobilising resources to help them deal with their problems.

For those service users who are clearly presenting with behaviours that are likely to need more specialist services and possible medication, a referral to the GP and then to psychiatric services would be appropriate and even necessary.

Diagnosis

A diagnosis of mental disorder is always given by a doctor who is usually also a psychiatrist. It emerges out of considerable contact between the doctor and the service user. Assessment as described above is a process of collecting information that will assist in the making of a diagnosis. Conventionally the language of psychiatry replaces 'mental disorder' with the term 'mental illness' and 'service user' with 'patient'. Psychiatrists are trained to use a phenomenological approach, or in other words they try to establish a pattern of signs and symptoms. This helps to distinguish between people who are eccentric, unusual or who have only occasional symptoms from those whose symptoms indicate more severe disorder.

To avoid variation in assessment between doctors it is common to use one of a number of psychiatric assessment tools or interview schedules. These have all been standardised, a process by which the reliability of these tools is established. They help the psychiatrist to assess the presence of certain symptoms which act as signposts to effective diagnosis. The schedules include the **Present State Examination (PSE)**, which has 40 components to it, or the more commonly used **Beck Depression Inventory.**

The importance of a diagnosis is that it:

- acts as a pathway to more specialised care and treatment;

- is a process in which most patients have faith (sometimes in spite of the evidence);

- can mobilise support from other agencies such as housing and income benefit for those in need;

- should involve other professional views being sought, including those of social workers;

- should occur over a period of time and not be an assessment that is made over a few days, but rather weeks or even months.

However, service users seldom report the diagnostic process as being empowering and often complain that their views are seldom sought except as signposts to a diagnosis.

Classification of mental disorders

Classification is an important step in the diagnosis of mental disorder. Mental disorder is broken down into various classifications that represent groups or syndromes of symptoms or phenomena. Thus if a series of symptoms fits into a recognised pattern they can be classified as, for example, schizophrenia and a diagnosis made. A diagnosis is a short-hand version of what the psychiatrist believes to be wrong with the patient. Such classifications also enable treatment and outcomes to be better predicted. In the UK psychiatrists use one of two texts, either the **DSM-IV** (American Psychiatric Association's Diagnostic and Statistical Manual of Mental disorders) or the **ICD-10** (International Classification of Diseases Volume 10 (World Health Organisation, 1992)). Although as a social worker you will not be using these to diagnose it is worth familiarising yourself with some of the main features. This will help you to understand the basis of a diagnosis.

The nature of this process is rigorous and great efforts have been made to try to ensure their validity and reliability. For example the ICD, published in 1992, took nine years to prepare and was tested and included extensive field trials of the draft text in many countries

(Eldergill, 1997). Even so they have been the subject of dispute over the years (Menninger, 1963) and remember that a diagnosis is only as good as the information on which it is based. You might want to think about how much these diagnoses are affected by social factors, societal values and historical context.

Although as a social worker you are usually not directly involved with the determination of a diagnosis, you will need to share the ownership of it when working as part of a multi-disciplinary team. It is important that you have some understanding, at least of the main characteristics of the above and what the various treatment options are for each. You are also, more than most professionals, going to be involved in the complex interaction of the service user and their cultural and social background. For example with disorders like depression, which has a biological component to it, a combination of medication and social intervention is often the most effective treatment.

Treatment

There are different ways of treating users who have mental disorder. The effectiveness of such treatment depends upon the nature of the disorder and the skills of the people who are providing the treatment. These treatments are briefly discussed below. Every treatment option must have the risks weighed up alongside the possible benefits, for no treatment is without some cost and risk. Medical practitioners are trained first and foremost to do no harm to their patients. The dominant mode of treatment is medication but treatment also includes the following:

Psychosurgery
This is little used and then only for those with chronic conditions of obsessional and depressive disorders. It can only be given with the patient's informed consent, and Section 57 of the Mental Health Act (1983) applies to both informal and formal patients and pro-vides additional safeguards. This is irreversible removal or destroying of brain tissue.

Electroconvulsive therapy (ECT)
ECT consists of administering an electric shock to patients who are sedated and is usually used when there has been an inadequate response to medication. It can be an effective treatment for depression, especially when this is accompanied by psychotic delusions. Patients are usually given a course of treatment of six to 12 applications.

Psychological
Psychological inputs are many and varied and include:

- behavioural therapy which is based on learning theory;
- cognitive therapy which focuses on incorrectly learned behaviours;
- counselling which also has numerous variants;
- psychotherapy which also includes many variants;
- family therapy.

Alternative medicine

As yet many of the 'alternative therapies', although popular with service users, are not 'proven' by research. They include hypnotherapy, dance, acupuncture and herbal remedies, and can have a role to play in combination with other modes of treatment. As interest continues some clinical trials have suggested that for moderate depression St John's Wort may be effective, and evidence suggests that exercise may also perform a valuable function.

Medication

Medication has become an important part of the treatment of mental disorder for many service users but it is not the only way of managing mental disorder. Medication works by either stopping the release of chemicals in the brain or by increasing the activity of certain parts of the brain. In the 1950s there was a 'pharmacological revolution' with the arrival of new forms of medical treatment including Chlorpromazine (Jones, 1993). This changed the lives of many patients with enduring mental illness in long-stay hospitals by giving them the opportunity to be treated in the community.

Today there is a 'new revolution' of 'atypical' anti-psychotic drugs, which have far fewer side effects than the previous ones and are also in many instances more effective. Some of the older medications caused amenorrhoea in women, which may have prevented long-term users from having children, whereas the main side effect of the new medication is significant weight gain.

Medication is divided into six types:

Type	Example	Typical use
Anti-psychotics	Chlorpromazine, Risperidone and in treatment-resistant conditions Clozapine	Schizophrenia
Anti-depressants	Prozac (fluoxetine)	Depression
Anti-manic	Lithium	Mania
Anti-epileptic	Carbamazepine	Epilepsy
Anxiolytics	Diazepam	Anxiety states
Hypnotics	Temezepam	Insomnia

RESEARCH STATISTICS

Over the past decade the number of prescription items for anti-depressant drugs dispensed in England has more than doubled, from 9 million items in 1991 to 24 million in 2001. The cost of anti-depressant drugs dispensed in the community in England was £342 million in 2001.

(1991 to 2001: Social Trends 33)

Understanding the major forms of mental disorder

The dilemma facing anyone who works with disturbed people is to be able to differentiate between 'normal' and 'abnormal' behaviour. The unusual behaviour or eccentricities of people are what make life so interesting and we should value such diversity. Clearly though there is a point beyond which the eccentric becomes markedly disordered and the person is in need of help. The main disorders that you will come across are described in the next part of this chapter.

Schizophrenia

Schizophrenia is a complex disorder with a number of variants, although the prognosis is well understood by specialists. It is a neuropsychiatric disorder where a number of factors may have impacted upon the central nervous system and which results in a cluster of symptoms that are classified as schizophrenia. It is commonly thought, incorrectly, by the general public to be associated with dangerousness and extreme madness and thus carries a stigma which other diagnoses do not (Eldergill, 1997).

Symptoms can include the following.

Hallucinations
These are problems to do with sensory perception, which are real for the person who experiences them. They include: auditory hallucinations (including hearing voices) and somatic hallucinations (the user believes that they are experiencing phenomena like electricity running through their body).

Delusions
These are beliefs which are considered bizarre, are clearly not supported by the available evidence yet are held in an unshakable manner by the person. Delusions can be part of systematic thought or appear to be completely random. These are usually culturally specific, hence in the UK some people are deluded into grandiose thinking, believing that they are related to the royal family or are relatives of the prime minister.

Interference with thought
Thought insertion is a form of delusion involving the belief that someone else's thoughts can be placed in the person's mind. This can also be perceived as a form of thought control where it is believed that someone outside is controlling your thoughts, or thought broadcast where you believe that your private thoughts are being broadcast to the general public.

Schizophrenia affects about 1% of the population. The onset is usually during adolescence or early adulthood but can occur later on in life. Before an accurate diagnosis is made the symptoms should have been noted over at least six months and must include at least one active psychotic phase. Early recognition and treatment significantly improves the overall prognosis for the user, consequently social workers should be aware of this and raise this diagnosis as a possibility rather than waiting to see. Early medication can alter the course of schizophrenia (Frangou and Bryne, 2000).

Features associated with schizophrenia

Episodes may consist of three phases in which 'normal functioning' is interrupted as follows:

1. **Pre-onset or prodromal phase** in which noticeable changes occur including social isolation, difficulty in functioning, odd behaviour, blunted affect, bizarre ideas, and lack of energy. Friends and relatives may describe the person's behaviour during this phase as 'he/she is not the same person as they were'.

2. **Onset or active phase** is where the behaviours and thoughts are acutely psychotic and often include delusions, which are false or irrational beliefs; hallucinations in which the most common is hearing voices; incoherence; belief that others can read your mind or hear your innermost thoughts and feelings of persecution. These need to be present for at least a week and can be the result of some stressful psychosocial event.

3. **Residual phase** is very similar to the pre-onset phase except that the person may experience negative affect and a flattening of emotions. They could still be hearing voices or other psychotic features but these are less strong.

Treatment and management

The usual treatment regime is a combination of medication and psychosocial interventions. While medication does not 'cure' it can dramatically correct serious and abnormal phenomena such as hallucinations or delusions.

The over-representation of young Afro-Caribbean males who are diagnosed as having schizophrenia is of major concern and points to the lack of culturally sensitive practice (see Chapter 1).

What is the social work role?

Social work intervention can include:

- education with the service user and their family;
- helping to arrange appropriate low stress accommodation;
- networking with the service user to provide community support;
- the use of behavioural techniques to modify behaviours;
- encouraging compliance with medication;
- acting as an advocate for the service user where appropriate.

What is the outlook or prognosis for people with schizophrenia?

About one-third of people who are diagnosed with schizophrenia will completely recover but for the remainder the outlook is one that will include at least one more episode, and for some schizophrenia will turn into a major challenge for them and their families or carers. The picture is much better than it was 20 years ago, in large part due to more effective interventions and the emergence of the newer anti-psychotic drugs that have fewer side effects than their predecessors.

(Chapter 6 has an illustrative example about schizophrenia).

Mood disorders: depression

Depression is a group of mental disorders that can affect many of us at some point in our lives. It can affect anyone, at any age, and is often overlooked among the very young and the elderly. Depression is a disorder characterised by mood change which explains why this disorder is termed a mood or affective disorder. There are different types of depression including manic depression, post-natal depression and clinical or major depression that affect about 3 – 4% of the population in any one year. More females are affected than males.

Depression is cateorised into three levels of severity: mild, moderate or severe. The ICD-10 is a good source for further information about these levels. However in essence the mild level allows users to receive treatment from their GPs and to continue with much of their lives; the moderate sees the user continuing their social, work or domestic lives with increased difficulty and with the severe it is unlikely that the user will be able to live a 'normal' life and suicide is a distinct risk.

Features associated with depression

Anyone can suffer from depression from time to time and it only becomes of clinical interest when the severity increases or the duration of the episode is longer than might be expected. Assessment is carried out using some psychiatric rating scales (Becks Depression Inventory).

Treatment and management

A range of treatments is possible depending upon the severity of the disorder. Among the treatments indicated are courses of anti-depressant medications, including the use of Prozac which interacts with the neuro-chemical pathways both in the brain and elsewhere in the body. The use of medication is often combined with psycho-social intervention to provide effective treatment. In severe depression it is important to take the risk of suicide seriously and to consult about risk with your medical colleagues. The user should always be asked about suicide, and where they exhibit plans for suicide or preoccupation with it then this should be seen as clear intent and action taken. (See Chapter 5 for an example on suicide.)

What is the social work role?

Social work interventions can include:

- identification of risk;

- management of risk;

- encouraging service users to take prescribed medication;

- individual counselling;

- cognitive behavioural therapy (CBT);

- referring for specialist psychotherapy;

- community networking.

Mood disorder: bipolar affective disorder (manic depression)

This is a disorder in which the person can feel intermittently depressed and occasionally elated. In the ICD mania and depression are cited as opposite ends of the same spectrum, hence the term bipolar. Mania is characterised by extreme elevation of mood and physical and mental energy and activity. It can exist in its own right (unipolar) but usually it is accompanied by at least one episode of depression. Because during mania the user believes that he/she is well, treatment is difficult and the social and financial consequences can be damaging as the person squanders their money or does other similar extravagances. Consequently hospital in-patient treatment may be required in order for the user's mood to return to normal.

The main medication is lithium although there are other medications available. This is a mood stabiliser that works by controlling the extent of racing thoughts rather than sedation, and although it takes a few days to work it does seem to prevent a swing into depression. It is particularly effective in the prevention of relapse among patients who have previously been diagnosed.

Dual diagnosis

The term dual diagnosis covers a spectrum of disorders that combine with mental disorder. While these can include mental disorder and learning disability they generally refer to mental disorder and substance abuse. This latter category has presented acute wards in hospitals with some of the most serious of challenges. In urban areas many of the patients admitted to hospital have experience of substance misuse, a habit which some try to continue while they are on the ward. The most common forms of misuse are drugs and alcohol.

The relationship between these conditions and the interactive effect are complex. These include:

• mental disorder that precipitated substance abuse;

• mental disorder which is worsened by the overlay of substance abuse;

• intoxication and/or substance abuse which results in psychological symptoms;

• withdrawal of substance abuse that results in psychiatric symptoms.

(Adapted from *Dual Diagnosis Good Practice Guide*, DoH, 2002)

Jacqui Smith, The Minister for Health, said in April 2002

> *All too often people with 'dual diagnosis' – the twin problems of severe mental illness combined with drug and alcohol problems – have fallen between two stools, and been unable to find the help that they need from either mental health or substance misuse services.*
> (Launch of the Acute In-Patient Care and Dual Diagnosis guidance, Jacqui Smith, 2002)

The National Office of Statistics demonstrated high levels of drug use in prisons, suggesting that 10% of remand prisoners had a moderate drug dependency, 40% had a severe dependency and among remand prisoners who were substance abusers over 75% had mental health problems (in *Dual Diagnosis Good Practice Guide*, 2002).

There is an increased risk of suicide for people with dual diagnosis and as substance misuse is becoming more common it should always be looked for in assessments. Treatment can involve motivational interviewing, assertive outreach, individual counselling and most importantly providing an integrated service. Associated with drug and alcohol abuse are increased physical health problems.

What is the social work role?
Social work interventions can include:

- identification of risk;

- management of risk;

- encouraging service users to take prescribed medication;

- cognitive behavioural therapy (CBT);

- community networking;

- liaison with other agencies and professionals.

Organic disorders

The organic disorders considered here are those associated with increasing age, most notably dementia. However don't forget that older people can also experience depression and other mental disorders in much the same way as their younger counterparts. The presence of depression in older people should be actively looked for and the person's presentation can mean that organic disorder is masked behind other mental disorders. For example approximately one person in five suffers from depression when they are over 60 and about one in ten actually develops depression after they have reached retirement age. There is a heightened risk of suicide among older people with depression.

Alzheimer's disease is a degenerative disease where the brain has been irreversibly damaged. Similar symptoms can also occur through excessive and prolonged consumption of alcohol or as a result of traumatic injury, a stroke or misuse of drugs. Sometimes the impairment can be acute and recovery is possible. In the case of Alzheimer's disease, which is considered to be a chronic condition, the brain progressively degenerates which results in impaired intellect, disorientation and eventually death.

Features associated with Alzheimer's
It is important to distinguish between the 'normal' effects of ageing and the development of a progressive disorder like Alzheimer's. We all suffer the loss of brain cells as we age but with this disorder cell loss is more rapid and profound than would be expected. The rate of degeneration does vary but it is usual for this to get more rapid as the disorder progresses.

Treatment and management
The early stages can be accompanied by depression, anxiety and severe sleep disturbance as the service user may have insight into the progressive nature of this disorder. Older people do better in familiar surroundings than in institutional care, but admission to residential care may be necessary where there is significant risk of self-neglect.

What is the social work role?

Social workers will work as part of a team that ideally will provide a system of care that encompasses the provision of support services of different kinds to the user and their carers, depending on their level of need. The social work role includes arranging welfare benefits, providing information and explanation of the user's situation to family, neighbours and others, arranging and financing social support systems and eventually specialist nursing care if necessary (Eldergill, 1997).

Critical psychiatry

While for the last fifty years the medical model has dominated the explanatory landscape there have been pockets of disaffection that have gained their followers. Among these several key names, themselves psychiatrists, are to be found including Thomas Szasz who in *The Myth of Mental Illness* was opposed to use of compulsion to treat people who in his view were struggling with problems of everyday life rather than some mental illness; Ronald Laing who saw the family and family power struggles accounting for much of what we call schizophrenia; and more recently a movement called 'Critical Psychiatry'. Psychiatrist Duncan Double is one of a small number of professionals who look beyond conventional explanations and treatment of people who have mental health problems.

Why is it that a movement called critical psychiatry can find favour? The answer lies in part in the general need by the public and professionals alike to examine alternatives to conventional treatments of a range of health problems. The increased use of supplements to assist diet, the use of acupuncture and homeopathy all stand testimony to the general dissatisfaction with the increased technical and scientific focus of medicine in general and by inference psychiatry. They do not absolutely reject the use of medication but rather put medication into a range of treatments rather than, as it sometimes is seen, as the only treatment.

The fundamental tenet of critical psychiatry is to challenge the evidence base and in so doing inevitably to look at the psycho-social aspects of the service users life. Phil Thomas, a Consultant Psychiatrist puts this over very succinctly on the critical psychiatry website www.critpsynet.freeuk.com/

> *Critical psychiatry is part academic, part practical. Theoretically it is influenced by critical philosophical and political theories, and it has three elements. It challenges the dominance of clinical neuroscience in psychiatry (but does not exclude it); it introduces a strong ethical perspective on psychiatric knowledge and practice; it politicises mental health issues. Critical psychiatry is deeply sceptical about the reductionist claims of neuroscience to explain psychosis and other forms of emotional distress. It follows that we are sceptical about the claims of the pharmaceutical industry for the role of psychotropic drugs in the 'treatment' of psychiatric conditions. Like other psychiatrists we use drugs, but we see them as having a minor role in the resolution of psychosis or depression. We attach greater importance to dealing with social factors, such as unemployment, bad housing, poverty, stigma and social isolation. Most people who use psychiatric services regard these factors as more important than drugs. We reject the medical model in psychiatry and prefer a social model, which we find more appropriate in a multi-cultural society characterised by deep inequalities.*

In a forthcoming book Double explains that the main aim of Critical Psychiatry is to develop a more open approach to psychiatry and that professionals like social workers need to remain sceptical about the claims that drug companies make for the efficacy of their products. This is not about ignoring the advances and assistance that medication has made but more about seeing this as only one component of the toolkit. (*Critical Psychiatry: Limits of Madness,* 2006)

To work in a truly empowering way can run counter to the imposition of a biomedical regime in which it is possible to see control and restraint as dominant features rather than enabling and understanding. It is important to understand the cultural context in which service users experience mental health problems and the role that poverty, poor housing and oppression play in someone's mental health. This is where the alternative explanation called the Social Model needs consideration.

The social model

The social model fits well with the general holistic approach of social work and is the underlying rationale for mental health social work although it is by no means as influential as the medical model. Nevertheless there are numerous examples of practice where the social model underpins effective practice (Ramon, 2001; Tew, 2002).

There are several different perspectives even within this model:

- social causation;
- labelling;
- critical theory;
- social constructivism; and
- social realism.

Whereas the conventional medical approach puts illness down to genetics, viruses or some other biomedical cause, the social model looks at social and environmental causes. The implications of the medical model are that illness *is* a matter of bad luck and one that needs an individual reaction, whereas the social model highlights the social causes and hence invites social reaction. This latter approach brings into play issues of power, oppression and social exclusion (Tew, 2002).

Social causation

Social causation is a particular perspective that helps us to understand the interaction between social disadvantage and mental disorder. A psychiatric diagnosis is largely accepted and the interest of the sociologist is in the effect that societal inequalities and social exclusion have had on the person's mental health. Other variables such as gender, ethnicity and class can be incorporated into this explanatory model.

The concentration of people who are diagnosed as having schizophrenia in inner city areas is an interesting example of this perspective. For although it is a 'fact' that the incidence of schizophrenia in inner city areas is much higher than in the suburbs and that schizophrenia is predominantly a lower class disorder, this is far from being a causal relationship.

ACTIVITY *2.2*

What factor do you think could explain the concentration of people with schizophrenia in inner city areas? Write down your ideas.

There are many possibilities but among those in the literature are:

- The drift theory, in which people who are long-term sufferers of schizophrenia migrate from rural areas into cities where they can blend in more easily and where services are more likely to be concentrated. People with schizophrenia from upper classes may find that the debilitating effect of this disorder results in them being unable to maintain their position in society and a downward drift into the lower classes occurs.

- Alternatively it could be that being in poverty in cities is harder and more alienating for people and that this could result in increased incidences of the disorder.

Labelling theory

Perhaps one of the most influential theories is labelling theory which describes a process by which '**primary deviance**' occurs, such as strange behaviour which continues to be interpreted as mental disorder or '**secondary deviance**'.

Primary deviance, or the initial concerning behaviour, may not always be recognised as a mental disorder as people often explain this initial deviance in terms of everyday behaviour. Thus the person with a drinking problem may be tolerated by their partner who has convinced himself or herself that their behaviour is just another way of letting off steam, or the more bizarre behaviour may be dismissed as humorous. Pilgrim and Rogers (1999) describe this as the 'clinical iceberg' (p.13) with many symptoms missed when doctors making diagnoses explain behaviours outside the norm for that person in terms of what should be rather than what is, happening.

Secondary deviance occurs when the diagnosis is made and the person takes on, or is seen to have taken on, the deviant role. In the same way that in primary deviance some behaviour gets interpreted as 'usual' then some of the deviant behaviour also is seen as what is typical of a mentally disordered person. The sociologist Erving Goffman (1961) describes this as the making of a psychiatric patient and writes about the role that the hospital plays as a total institution.

Psycho-social causes of mental disorder

The early part of this chapter concentrated on the medical model in which work with service users is focused upon trying to identify the cause of the mental disorder in order that we can intervene to restore better mental health. We then briefly looked at the social model and now need to see how these two models can be applied to everyday practice. Most professionals accept that the most likely cause of mental disorder is a complex interaction between a range of factors and that we need to find a way of encompassing biological, psychological and social factors that may be present. Newton (1988) is one of many academics who have constructed models that not only help us to see possible causes, but also to identify what might be done with the service user to improve their functioning.

A simplified version of these models is set out in Figure 2.1 and shows how factors can interact with each other to determine whether in any given circumstance a person will develop either good or poor mental health. These factors are:

- Predisposing or vulnerability factors including genetic components and previous family or personal history of mental health problems.

- Social causative factors including the importance of class, social exclusion and racism in reinforcing mental disorder.

- Psychological factors including loss, threats, highly critical relationships, resilience to adverse events and the extent of social support networks that precipitate or trigger the onset of disorder.

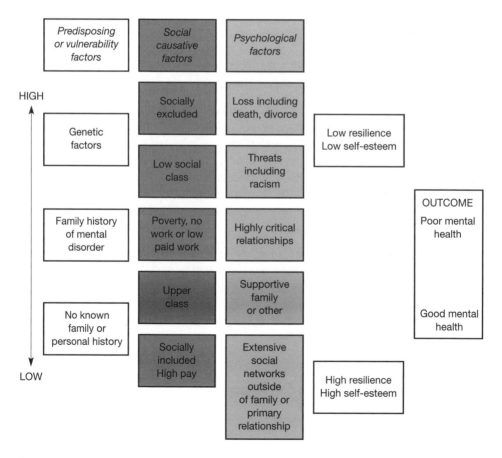

Figure 2.1: *Psycho-social model*

It is important that you realise that these models are an oversimplification of complex situations and that different authors use different terminology. Nevertheless they at least provide an indication of where people might be vulnerable and offer the possibility of intervention to help strengthen the weak areas.

This approach allows you to weigh up the factors and with the service user to work out what could be achieved to promote their mental good health. It also helps explain how people can face similar events but react differently. Thus although the service user may have a history of family mental health problems, they may be in a well-paid, satisfying job and with a network of social support. These factors could interact to provide protective rather than vulnerability factors. Of course the opposite might occur where no previous history of mental disorder is known but social exclusion and the resultant stress may increase the person's vulnerability to mental health problems.

Social work practice in a psycho-social context

The reality of intervening in people's lives is that you are working with something that is complex and multifaceted (O'Sullivan, 1999). At the centre of our work is helping service users to manage their lives in ways that are better for them and for their families and society. Any intervention carries with it a degree of uncertainty about the effect that this intervention might have on the service user.

The present drive to integrate services for people with mental disorder in theory opens up the opportunity to provide a seamless service. Social workers will work alongside health colleagues and it will be obvious to both just what they each bring to the situation. The need for quality evidence on which to support the specific intervention is long overdue and the establishment of centres for evidence-based practice (Huxley, 2002, p.198) suggests that social care is beginning to embrace the idea of measuring changes that have occurred as a result of their and others' interventions.

The Cochrane Centre provides systematic reviews of the effects of health care interventions and has a number of mental health groups in the collaboration, all of which can be accessed through their website: www.cochrane.org. The evidence that we have already shows that psycho-social intervention can have a powerful effect on rehabilitation; respite care to relieve the impact on carers can delay hospitalisation; family interventions can alleviate some of the negative aspects of living with someone who has mental disorder; intervention aimed at improving the living environment and creating or supporting social networks is effective; family work can be effective in reducing the emotionally charged and overly-critical family environments.

What works less well appears to be psychological debriefing after trauma, crisis intervention and case management (Huxley, 2002).

Examine Figure 2.1 and refer to either a case study that you know or one that is in this book. Lisa's story in Chapter 4 would work well for this activity.

Break down the case study into the factors that fit into this diagram and weight them according to your assessment of the likelihood of them increasing vulnerability or protecting against vulnerability to poor mental health.

You do not have enough detailed information to fully complete this task and that is perhaps the first important point to learn – analysis of causes is complex and requires careful collection of the 'evidence'.

The evidence that you have may well point to consideration of some of the factors such as does the service user belong to a black and minority ethnic group and if so is this likely to make them more vulnerable or less vulnerable? Similarly are they socially excluded? Is their financial situation stable?

If you work from right to left when looking at Figure 2.1 you should be able to get some idea of how various factors can interact to produce either a positive outcome or a negative one:

- **Predisposing or vulnerability factors** e.g. family with a history of mental disorder would make you more vulnerable to developing mental disorder.

- **Social causative factors** e.g. being unemployed or socially excluded (such as asylum seekers).

- **Psychological factors** e.g. no supportive relationships.

All of these factors could interact to produce low resilience, low self-esteem and therefore an increased likelihood of poor mental health.

You might want to think about what would have to change to increase resilience. A note of caution is needed, as it is unlikely that relationships between these factors would be simple or straightforward.

Stress is an intervening variable

Of course you probably realise that people experience similar events differently, the loss of job to one person could be a crushing blow that results in a vulnerability to depression yet to another it could be the very opportunity to go to college to get better qualified or to just take some time out. This will almost certainly be influenced by previous experience, family circumstances and financial position.

Epstein (1983) suggests that it is possible to learn better ways of coping with stress while writers like Cochrane (1983) point to the role that stress plays in pushing people either towards positive mental health or in the other direction. It is not just the experience of losing your job but the way in which this impacts upon you and, importantly, how you perceive the event. This approach does open up the prospect of working with the service user to recognise what makes them overstressed and to identify better ways to manage their stress. It is clearly not possible to reduce all the adverse events that affect a person's life but it is possible to get better at managing the situations that might cause them and their reactions to them.

EXAMPLE

Social workers working with families and young people who are on the road to recovery from an eating disorder can do work on some of the factors that cause the service user to feel under pressure about their eating habits, Among these short-term techniques are included:

- *not asking about what person has eaten;*
- *avoiding making comments about the food;*
- *not making comments about shape or size;*
- *not telling them that they look good or healthy;*
- *not making any comments about their weight.*

This puts the consideration of weight and size into the professional domain and removes everyday comments from family members that may be considered stressful.

Promoting mental well-being: a political approach

Newton provides information about what is needed to provide the necessary conditions to prevent mental disorder. Two possible approaches to prevention are either to work to reduce the vulnerability factors, or helping people to develop more positive responses and increased resilience to withstand stressful situations. It is a political approach as many of the social factors include the effects of social exclusion, racism and poverty.

Work that falls into the category of reducing vulnerability would include social workers being placed in schools and projects with specific funding, such as Sure Start. In both instances the work can be focused upon the young person and their families. Some of the work compensates for social disadvantage and could have a positive impact on mental health.

Promoting positive mental health: saving lives

Our Healthier Nation (1999) was a direct attempt by government to create a healthier nation by reducing the incidence of mental disorder. In 2003 the then Minister for Health Jacqui Smith launched England's first ever national suicide prevention strategy. It is hoped that by identifying key factors that are associated with suicide such deaths could be significantly reduced.

ACTIVITY 2.4

Go back to Figure 2.1 and think where would be the best focus for a suicide prevention strategy. What factor would make people more vulnerable to suicide thoughts? Jot down your ideas.

You probably came up with most of the factors that are identified in the policy document. These would include people who are:

- in low paid, unskilled work;

- unemployed;

- breaking up from their relationship;

- socially isolated;

- misusing drugs or alcohol.

Having an impact in all these areas would help and we do not actually know which one would make the biggest difference. This requires a mixture of social policy and community initiatives.

Equally, working with service users who are depressed to improve their social networks would help, and so would encouraging service users to continue taking their medication.

Despite the methodological problems the government has moved forward with its intentions to affect the number of suicides with year-on-year reductions set as targets. Progress is being made but even so over 1,300 young adult men take their own lives each year in England, a number which has now overtaken road deaths as the biggest killer of young men in this age category (Brock and Griffiths, 2003). Overall over 4,500 people take their own lives each year. Some of the actions that have been taken include:

- Reducing the pack sizes of aspirin and paracetamol in an attempt to make it more difficult for people to purchase large quantities of these tablets.

- Improving the risk assessment on inpatient wards where acute patients are liable to be detained.

- Establishing a research forum to improve the quality of the information that is available to professionals to ensure that professional practice is evidence based.

- Working more closely with service user groups.

- Setting up a number of pilot projects to target key at-risk groups such as young men.

With the last two actions social workers will be among the key professionals who will help to put these initiatives into operation.

It is too early to comment authoritatively about the effectiveness of this plan and authoritative evaluations are needed.

C H A P T E R   S U M M A R Y

This chapter has introduced you to the two main theoretical approaches to understanding mental health. As required by the subject benchmark you should have developed your knowledge of the critical and research-based explanations that contribute to the knowledge base of social work, including the application to practice. As a social worker you need to have at least a basic understanding of the medical model and the major mental illnesses that can affect service users. This will enable you to have more meaningful dialogue with medical colleagues and to work in an informed way with service users.

Detail has been provided about mental disorder, intervention and treatment. Included in this has been a description of the main types of medication that are currently in use, and all this should help you to feel more confident and knowledgeable about mental health. The role of social workers in working with people who have mental disorder or mental health problems has been outlined and the provision of a schematic outline of psychosocial factors will help you to see where the best intervention ought to be made. As this model underpins most of social work practice when working with people who have mental health problems, it will be referred to over the next chapters.

In-depth case studies are provided in later chapters that build up your specific knowledge of depression, schizophrenia and eating disorders.

Stress busting tip

Preventing stress and promoting positive mental health by developing an effective support system

As you have seen in this chapter stress can play a large part in our mental health and can trigger mental health problems and disorder. Having a support system that provides support for you can help you and others to deal effectively and more healthily with stress. This support can be informal or formal, the key is what works for you. What does help is being able to talk things through with someone who helps you to see the positive side of things and can help you to construct solutions rather than dwelling upon the problems. This should help you to move into a 'glass half full' perspective rather than a 'glass half empty' one.

Consider your own support systems. If possible find a friend and go through this list recording your answers. The content of the discussion is confidential to you and you should only discuss what you feel comfortable with.

Support network

Do you currently have:

1. Someone on whom you can rely in a crisis?

2. Someone who makes you feel good about yourself?

3. Someone you can be totally yourself with?

4. Someone who will tell you, honestly, how well or badly you are doing?

5. Someone you can talk to if you are worried?

6. Someone who really makes you stop and think about what you are doing?

7. Someone who is lively to be with?

8. Someone who introduces you to new ideas, new interests, new people?

Of course to find all these 'ideal type' attributes in one person would be truly special and even if you did find such a person, putting all of this on them might be too much and put a strain on relationships. There are also key times when we may need extra support and have to either seek professional help or develop a new network.

If you have been able to reflect on this list you may now want to reflect a little more.

Is your support coming from one person? Is this from home or student life? Do you need a better balance between these two? What gaps have you got in your support network? What are you going to do about these gaps? If you have more gaps than you would like, work out how to alter this – you may want to find someone who can help you, perhaps a student counsellor.

FURTHER READING

Anselm Eldergill's, (1998) seminal work *Mental Health Review Tribunals: Law and practice* is a classic in its own right and a surprisingly rich source for anyone who wants to read in depth on the origins, causes and treatment of mental disorder. In the 300 pages devoted to these topics he shows a remarkable grasp of detail and an enviable ability to explain these to non-medics. His work has greatly influenced the content of this chapter.

D Pilgrim and A Rogers', (1999) *A Sociology of Mental Health and Illness* (2nd ed) is a best-selling text and one of a number of texts that illustrate the key perspectives on mental health. It has good chapters on social class inequalities and mental health, gender, race and ethnicity and age, all of which make for interesting and relevant reading.

WEBSITES

Social Trends can be downloaded free from www.statistics.gov.uk

Chapter 3
The legal and policy context

This chapter will help you to begin to meet the following National Occupational Standards:

Key Role 1: Prepare for and work with individuals, families, carers, groups and communities to assess their needs and circumstances

- Assess needs and options to recommend a course of action.

Key Role 2: Plan, carry out, review and evaluate social work practice, with individuals, families, carers, groups and communities and other professionals

- Interact with individuals, families, carers, groups and communities to achieve change and development and to improve life opportunities.
- Address behaviour which presents a risk to individuals, families, carers, groups and communities.

It will also introduce you to the following academic standards as set out in the social work subject benchmark statement, which includes:

2.2.2 Defining principles

There are competing views in society at large of the nature of social work and its place and purpose. Social work practice and education inevitably reflect these differing perspectives on the role of social work in relation to social justice, social care and social order.

3.1.1 Social work services and service users

- The nature and validity of different definitions of, and explanations for, the characteristics and circumstances of service users and the services required by them.

3.1.4 Social work theory

- Research-based concepts and critical explanations from social work theory and other disciplines that contribute to the knowledge base of social work, including their distinctive epistemological status and application to practice.

The subject skills highlighted to demonstrate this knowledge in practice include:

- Assessing human situations, taking into account a variety of factors.
- Assessing the merits of contrasting theories.

Introduction

The end of law is, not to abolish or restrain, but to preserve and enlarge freedom.
John Locke (1690)

The law concerning persons who suffer from mental disorder is a vast subject and practically every area of law makes some special provision for persons whose capacity or responsibility for their acts is impaired.
(Eldergill, 1998, p.4)

With the above quotes in mind this chapter concentrates upon the principles and practice of the main statutes that relate to mental health. These include the major provisions of the Mental Health Act, Code of Practice and Memorandum as they relate to the admissions process both civil and through the courts, detention in hospital, treatment in hospital and in the community, discharge and appeals processes. In order to work effectively in multi-disciplinary settings you need to have a broad knowledge of processes that will impact on service users with whom you work.

The government in March 2006 abandoned the long awaited Mental Health Bill. This was to have been the legislation that would 'modernise' the legal framework in which social work-ers and others operate. It was hugely controversial and met with opposition from a variety of professional bodies and user groups alike. As a consequence of this the government looked again at the argument for the Bill and what it was that they sought to achieve. Consequently we now await the introduction, when parliamentary time allows, of a much shorter and streamlined Bill that will amend the present 1983 Act.

However some of the more controversial elements such as compulsory treatment in the community will remain as one of the cornerstones of the government's attempts as they see it to promote service user safeguards, conform to the European Standards on Human Rights and to protect the public from harm.

Although every attempt has been made to guarantee accuracy there is no substitute for going back to first principles and reading the Mental Health Act and the Code of Practice, and remember – all legislation is experimental and subject to changing interpretations as case law builds up.

The term 'patient' is used in the legislation and for the most part by hospitals, and to avoid confusion this is the term that is used in this chapter.

The need for legislation?

Mental health and the law have in recent history been inextricably linked together.

ACTIVITY 3.1

Think about why people who have mental health problems should be subject to legisla-tion. Try to list at least three reasons.

You probably listed things such as that people who have mental health problems may pose a risk to themselves and others; they may need compulsory admission to hospital for treatment; they are incapable at times of consent even though they may be ill. Perhaps you had some more ideas as well.

There is a curious paradox operating here, which does not apply to any other area of health and social care. If you are mentally ill, something that no one can absolutely establish, you can be admitted to hospital against your wishes and be made to have treatment, even though you do not want it, which at best can only alleviate the symptoms. Compare that with someone who has pneumonia, which can be proven and in the vast majority of instances cured, but for which you cannot be made to go into hospital nor can you be forced to have treatment.

What explanation can be found that stands up to scrutiny and can justify such a position?

Tensions between public safety and individual freedom

Applications are seldom only for medical reasons and most applications are justified as necessary to protect the patient or the public from serious harm. Consequently the admissions process is never far away from considerations of risks and risk management.

Elsewhere the idea of developing culturally sensitive practice is covered (Chapter 1) and this is important to take into consideration. This includes social workers and other professionals being aware of the cultural and social context in which the patient is being assessed.

RESEARCH SUMMARY

The Department of Health publishes annual bulletins providing information about people detained in NHS facilities, including high security psychiatric hospitals and private mental nursing homes, under the 1983 Mental Health Act. These show among other statistics that the number of formal admissions to hospital under the Act rose from 16,000 in 1988–89 to 27,100 in 1998–99 and have remained steady from that date, and that 89% of all formal admissions were to NHS hospitals under Part II of the Act. (Statistical Bulletin 2002/26)

The framework for compulsory admission

The primary legislation is the **Mental Health Act 1983** as amended by the **Mental Health (Patients in the Community) Act 1995**. Guidance on this legislation can be found in the **Mental Health Act 1983: The Code of Practice (DoH,1999)**.

The Mental Health Act 1983 provides admission to and a means of discharge from hospital, an appeal process and, where appropriate, treatment and support in the community. The Act is made up of ten parts and numerous sections. Part I defines to whom this statute refers; Part II refers to compulsory admissions; Part III covers admission through the courts; Part IV covers treatment, etc. Within each part are sections which provide the detail; e.g.section 2 (s.2) refers to compulsory admission to hospital for assessment and section 41(s.41) lays down the restrictions that can be made by a Crown Court. There are key people who are involved in the process of compulsory admissions who are:

- the approved social worker;
- the nearest relative;
- the doctors;
- the hospital managers.

And, of course, the subject of the legislation – the patient.

Who is an approved social worker?

Under the Mental Health Act 1983 the Approved Social Worker must be an employee of the Local Authority Social Services Authority (s.114 (2)). The Director of Social Services must ensure that there are sufficient numbers of Approved Social Workers in their area (s.114(1)) and the General Social Care Council oversees the quality and type of training that the Approved Social Worker must undertake.

Although some writers trace the role of the Approved Social Worker back to the unpaid overseer of the poor under the 1601 Poor Law Relief Act this is slightly spurious and in practice the emergence of a specialist mental health worker is far more recent (Curran *et al.*, 1999). The present day Approved Social Worker emerged from the Mental Welfare Officer who has had the responsibility for arranging admission and the aftercare of service users since the NHS was established in 1948.

The Approved Social Worker is central to admissions process and a vital component of a mental health service. The tenth Biennial Report of the Mental Health Act Commission comments:

> *Social Workers who are approved under section 114 … undergo what is probably the most thorough training on the provisions of the Act currently available to any mental health professional.* (p.113)

As the move towards community based multi-disciplinary teams has gained momentum social workers have been transferred to local health care trusts. This has resulted in a confused situation in which such health trusts cannot employ ASWs as they need to be 'officers of the Local Authority'. The proposed amendment to the Act will most likely result in a new form of Approved Mental Health Professional who will replace the ASW. The government's proposals are hard to understand and worth closer examination. Hewitt has drawn our attention to the prime motives behind the government's intentions being (a) to update the principles and process and (b) to ensure that the knowledge base of the new Approved Mental Health Professional is more current (Hewitt, 2005, pp. 144–5)

This is strange as the principle behind the present Act is that the ASW is in effect representing the lay perspective or more appropriately the social model and this should be in a tension with the medical model that so features in psychiatry. So in future the new professional may not be a social worker and could conceivably be a nurse employed by the same trust as the patient is to be admitted to. In any event as Hewitt points out the loss of the

ASWs' much valued independence will not increase the confidence that service users have in the system. Although many ASWs now find themselves located in trusts they remain employees of the Local Authority.

This vital equilibrium as Peter Gilbert describes it is echoed by others and he presents a good argument for retaining this role as a social work one. In particular he draws upon Stanley and Manthorpe in their work on Mental Health Inquiries

> *The unique role of the ASW as the co-ordinator of assessments, a repository of legal and procedural knowledge represents a holistic, humanistic approach with an established commitment to anti-oppressive practice.*
> (Stanley and Manthorpe, 2001, p.96 in Gilbert 2003, p.72).

As Hewitt points out the arguments that Government have advanced to replace the ASW do not stack up and the present location of the ASW in many Trusts may paradoxically be an Approved Mental Health Professional in all but name (Hewitt, 2005, p.148). We will have to wait to see if the proposals come to the Statute and when the implementation date will be.

Although many aspects of working in this legal context have been given to the ASW it is important that all social workers have at the very least an overview of legal provisions and what the responsibilities are for the people involved. Mental disorder and mental health problems are so prevalent in society that most social workers will work with service users who experience these problems alongside the initial presenting problem. For example you may be working as a child protection worker and discover that the primary carer has long-term mental health problems. It is important to know what the ASW does.

What is the role of the Approved Social Worker?

The Approved Social Worker has duties and powers under the Act that include:

- Making the application.
- Conveying the patient to hospital.
- Taking patients who are absent without leave back to the hospital.
- Applying to a Justice of the Peace in the Magistrates' Court for a warrant to search for and remove patients believed to be suffering from a mental disorder, being ill treated, neglected, living alone or in need of care.
- Applying to the County Court to displace or to appoint a nearest relative.
- Interviewing a person removed by the police under Section 136 to a place of safety.
- Providing a social circumstances report for the patient's Mental Health Review Tribunal.
- Providing a written report to the hospital after each compulsory admission.
- Providing a written report including a recommendation that the grounds for aftercare under supervision have been met.

(Extract from Curran et al., 1995)

How is this duty exercised?

The Approved Social Worker is personally liable for his/her actions whilst carrying out the above functions. This requires that the ASW should exercise their judgement and not simply act under the direction of their employers, medical practitioners and others who are concerned with the care and treatment of the service user. There is protection for the ASW in the Act, providing that they have acted in a way that the courts would determine as being reasonable.

Working as a part of the assessment process while retaining independence is a difficult task and not without its problems. In 1957 the Percy Commission were clear that ... *no responsible mental welfare officer would lightly disregard or dissent from (a doctor's) advice ...* and it was only with the 1983 Act that the independence of the ASW role was confirmed as an important part of the decision-making process. There was considerable opposition at the time to this increased power, especially from the medical profession for whom this was largely a question of 'turf wars', but even within local authorities there was unhappiness at this level of independence and with it responsibility for training without additional financial resources.

Although much of this opposition has since evaporated it set the scene for difficult relationships between medical practitioners and social workers. Some social services have problems recruiting and retaining a 'sufficient number' of Approved Social Workers. At present in order to become an ASW many authorities require at least two years' post professional qualification and the successful completion of a 12-week training course. This is often followed by a period shadowing an experienced Approved Social Worker to develop competence in real life situations. This would appear to have had a good effect as recent research suggests that ASWs are sometimes able to make better judgements about a person's need for hospitalisation than their medical counterparts including the psychiatrist (Bartlett and Sandland, 2003).

Admission to hospital (Part II)

Admission to a psychiatric hospital is usually informal, sometimes called voluntary and is defined in s.131 of the MHA which applies to any person who is 16 years or older. It provides the same rights of discharge, and refusal of treatment that any patient in any hospital has under the common law. However should a patient try to discharge themselves and it is considered not appropriate they can be held in hospital (s.5). This allows either a prescribed nurse or doctor to hold the patient in hospital until such time as a more formal process of assessment followed by admission can be undertaken.

Where compulsory admission is necessary a rigorous approach to the legally driven process should be adopted. There is no lower or upper age limit imposed on persons who are subject to these provisions.

It is possible to think of mental health law as a wall that either stops you from getting into hospital or getting out.

The medical recommendations

This wall needs firm foundations and the first block is the medical recommendations. It is important to realise that this process does not involve the courts, except in specific circumstances.

Nature or degree of mental disorder

Two medical recommendations are used in the majority of cases, except where there is an emergency and getting two doctors would be very detrimental to either the service user or others. Both doctors should not have a personal interest in the patient and both must have examined the patient within prescribed time limits. One of the doctors should have specialised knowledge of mental disorder (a psychiatrist).

The medical recommendation is based on the identification of a legally classified form of mental disorder, not a medical diagnosis.

> *Mental disorder means mental illness, arrested or incomplete development of mind, psychopathic disorder and any other disorder or disability of mind.*
> (MHA, 1983,s.1(2))

Mental disorder is further broken down into four forms. These are:

- mental illness;

- severe mental impairment;

- mental impairment;

- psychopathic disorder.

Mental illness is not further defined although the majority of compulsory admissions occur within this category. The use of the general form allows disorders such as eating disorders to be included in the Act but it also carries the risk of including eccentric or bizarre behaviours. This legal form includes schizophrenia, mood disorders but excludes promiscuity, sexual deviancy or dependence upon alcohol or drugs. The difference between mental impairment and severe mental impairment is one of the degree of severity and both mean *a state of arrested or incomplete development of mind which includes significant impairment of intelligence that is associated with abnormally aggressive or seriously irresponsible conduct.* Psychopathic disorder, the subject of much controversy, means *a persistent disorder that results in abnormally aggressive or seriously irresponsible conduct* (MHAC s.1(2-3)).

The doctor should also assess the nature and degree of the person's mental state and the need for medical treatment in hospital. These recommendations, made by a doctor who will probably know the person and the other by a medical health specialist, provide the basic building blocks for the admission process (see below). Only when the medical recommendations are complete can the application be made by the ASW or nearest relative. The medical assessment is to determine if the patient is suffering from mental disorder that is sufficiently serious to make in-patient treatment or guardianship necessary. This consideration should be discussed with the applicant and the other doctor involved (unless it is an emergency admission when only one doctor is required) and if a recommendation for admission is made the doctor must ensure that a hospital bed is available.

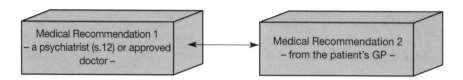

Health and safety and the protection of others

The presence of a serious mental disorder is by itself an insufficient a reason for compulsory admission as many disorders can be treated effectively within the community. Consequently the grounds for admission, once the presence of the legal classification of mental disorder is established, must include meeting the conditions that it must be for his/her own health or for his/her safety or for the protection of others. In the case of Guardianship 'health or safety' is replaced by the narrower concept of welfare. These are not further defined and interpretation by the professionals involved is needed.

Together these provide the foundation for an admission. On its own a medical recommendation is insufficient and the application must be made by either the Approved Social Worker or in a small number of cases by the nearest relative. The social worker must decide that, in all circumstances of the case, compulsory admission to hospital is the least restrictive of the alternatives to the person remaining in the community. It need not be the last resort but the social worker must come to an independent view that it is in all the circumstances the best option. Where appropriate a Guardianship order (s. 7) should be considered.

The application

The application can only be made if it is on the foundation of medical assessment. The ASW is expected to have an opinion that is separate from, but informed by, the medical view. In recent years evidence has begun to build up that ASWs are playing an important independent role in this process, exercising a more holistic view that takes into account issues about social context and culture, as well as being in the best position to mobilise community support systems. The application must be made on the prescribed statutory form and be accepted by the hospital.

> Social workers provide a safeguard against unnecessary use of compulsory powers by bringing a balancing, non-medical view of the best interests of the patient and the need to use the least restrictive option available to provide care.
> (Tenth Biennial Report, 8.75, p.113)

We now have the two-stage procedure complete and, when all parties agree, the process of compulsory admission to hospital can get underway.

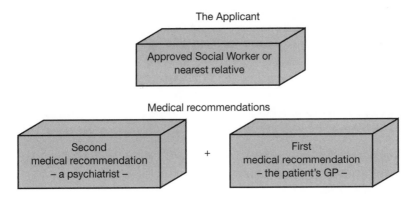

Once the application has been made to the managers of the hospital (s.11 MHA 1983) there is a power to convey the patient to hospital. This usually means arranging for an ambulance and the Approved Social Worker following the ambulance to the hospital.

ACTIVITY **3.2**

Imagine that a service user and family have asked you to explain the process of civil compulsory admission. Try to do this – say it out loud and then check it out against the previous pages.

The applicant: nearest relative or Approved Social Worker?

Although we have described the role of the Approved Social Worker (ASW), the nearest relative (NR) in consultation with the ASW can also act as the applicant. The nearest relative is defined in the Act in s.26 (see Glossary).The Code of Practice recommends that the Approved Social Worker should be the applicant of choice, recognising the potential adverse impact on the relationship between the nearest relative and the patient. Where the nearest relative wishes to proceed with the admission the social services must supply a social circumstances report to the admitting hospital and it is the duty of the hospital to notify the area social services department of any such admissions (MHA 1983, s.14). It may seem strange that specific training is required of ASWs while for the nearest relative there is no similar requirement or even expectation of any knowledge about mental health.

If the ASW is the applicant, and they are for over 90% of all applications, they shall take all reasonable steps to ensure that the nearest relative is informed of any decision to admit a patient to hospital. The nearest relative can object and in so doing prevent the admission process from continuing. If this objection is considered to be against the best interests of the patient the ASW can seek to displace the nearest relative in favour of themselves through an application to the courts.

Assessments for admission should involve professionals with different perceptions coming to a common view that admission to hospital is in all circumstances the most appropriate action to be taken. However Bowers *et al.* (2003) observes that this can be a rather instrumental approach and largely one in which the main challenge is to get all the 'agents' together at the right time rather than resolving deep professional and philosophic differences.

Susan is a young woman, aged 28 and a single parent, who has a history of manic depression and has been detained many times in the local psychiatric hospital. Although compliant with care plans she will not entertain the idea of going into hospital on an informal or voluntary basis. She usually remains in hospital for about two weeks before returning home to care for her three children. She lives in poor accommodation and has few links with her ethnic community who have largely abandoned her to her own devices.

Consider the options that ought to be available for Susan. How do these options compare with your knowledge of local services?

Admissions like this are referred to as 'revolving door'. You need to consider the extent that this represents the form of mental disorder that Susan experiences or the influence that social factors have had on her and her family. The impact upon her children and their care needs careful consideration (see Chapter 7).

What if Susan did not speak English as her first language? You would need to obtain the services of an interpreter.

Trained mental health interpreter

If the patient is mentally ill and not English speaking it is essential that the Approved Social Worker and other health care professionals involved in their detention under the 1983 MHA give them the opportunity to communicate effectively. It is worth remembering that the patient may be about to lose his/her freedom for 28 days to six months. Therefore where the patient and/or their NR is assessed as being unable to speak fluent English, the hospital or social services should always ensure that a trained interpreter (language or signing) is available.

Compulsory admission criteria

The following chart describes the basic criteria that need to be met for the most common sections that are used to admit someone to hospital.

Capacity

An individual may lose their ability to make decisions in a wide range of circumstances. For example, an elderly person with dementia or an individual in an acute stage of their mental illness may be unable to make decisions for themselves. This inability is sometimes referred to as a loss of capacity. This loss may be temporary or permanent or may fluctuate. Whatever the circumstances, health and social care professionals need to ensure that individuals who lack capacity are protected from exploitation and their autonomy and dignity are maintained as far as possible. It is presumed in English law that an adult has full capacity unless it can be shown that s/he does not and new legislation was introduced in 2005 to establish a test of capacity. A person has capacity if s/he can understand and retain the information relevant to the decision in question, can believe that information and can assess it in arriving at a choice. Most people, even at times of severe mental distress are able to make some decisions for themselves. Although their level of capacity may vary significantly over a period of time, there may be lucid intervals where the individual regains their ability to act.

	Section 2	Section 3	Section 4
Duration up to	Assessment (includes treatment): 28 days cannot be renewed	Treatment: six months initially, then for a further six months, then periods of one year	Emergency 72 hours
Application by	ASW or NR	ASW or NR	ASW or NR
Criteria (see appropriate section in the MHA, 1983)	Mental disorder (not specified)	Specified as one of the four classifications	Mental disorder and urgent necessity Can be 'converted' to a s.2 with additional recommendation
Medical recommendation	Two recommendations	Two recommendations	One recommendation
Mental Health Review Tribunal	Yes, within 14 days	Yes, once in first six months and once in each subsequent period of detention	No
Hospital Managers' Review	Yes	Yes	Yes
Discharge by	RMO, NR, MHRT or Hospital Managers' Review (HMR)	RMO, NR, MHRT or Hospital Managers' Review	RMO or HMR

(Adapted from Curran *et al*. (2002))

Best interests

Decisions made on behalf of a person without capacity should be made in their best interests. The 1983 Mental Health Act Revised Code of Practice recommends that if a patient lacks capacity at the time of an assessment for admission to hospital or a review, it is particularly important that both clinical and social care requirements are considered and that account is taken of the patient's ascertainable wishes and feelings and the views of their immediate relatives and carers on what would be in the patient's best interests.

The assumption made is that the patient has the capacity to understand what is happening to them and in particular is able to understand the implications of treatment and to consent or not to the treatment. There are few instances in physical medicine where the refusal of treatment can be overridden. If they are detained under the MHA (1983) the patient's right to refuse can be set aside providing the correct procedure is followed.

Advance directives

Individuals, aged 18 or over, who have the mental capacity (see *Openmind* July/August No 98, p.24) may state that they want to refuse certain treatments in advance so that their wishes are respected at a later date if they lose their capacity or cannot communicate for some reason. These statements may be referred to in a number of ways, for example, 'living wills', 'advance directives', 'advance statements', or 'advance refusals'. The law recognises that a mentally capable adult can refuse treatment, even if that refusal leads to deterioration in their condition or may indeed be fatal. By leaving clear instructions, an individual can make treatment choices in the event that capacity is lost. To be valid and therefore legally enforceable, an advance refusal of treatment must be available to the treatment provider and must be clear, unambiguous and cover the treatment now proposed. In the case of detained patients they can be overridden by the MHA without going to court. If there is doubt then an application to the courts may be considered for a declaration that the proposed treatment is lawful, with clinically appropriate treatment being provided in the interim.

Short-term powers

There are powers to respond to people who are in a public place and may be exhibiting mental disorder or who are believed to have mental disorder but are refusing access to where they reside.

Police holding power under s.136

If a person who is in a public place is suspected of being mentally disordered they can be removed by the police using the powers of s.136 to enable them to be examined by a doctor and interviewed by an Approved Social Worker (ASW), and for suitable arrangements to be made for their care and treatment. It may also provide an appropriate means of diversion from the criminal justice system.

The term 'public place' covers any place to which the public has access, e.g. a public highway, railway platform or hospital casualty department. Although a hospital is the preferred 'place of safety', it may also be: [i] local authority residential accommodation; [ii] a police station; [iii] an independent mental health hospital/care home; or [iv] any other suitable place. Consideration should be given to the possible impact of the place of safety upon the assessment process e.g. members of some minority ethnic groups may consider police stations threatening.

Once the patient arrives at the place of safety, the removed person may be detained there and only there for up to 72 hours. The authority for detention under s.136 will, however, expire immediately the assessment process has been completed, even if this is within 72 hours. The police have primary responsibility for liaison in s.136 cases. If the place of safety is a hospital, they should contact the local social services department [SSD]; if a police station, they should also contact the appropriate doctor (e.g. forensic medical examiner or psychiatrist). The SSD should in turn ensure that an ASW attends as soon as possible.

HISTORICAL NOTE

The origins of s.136 lie in the Vagrancy Acts of 1714 and 1744, which empowered magistrates to order the detention of a `lunatic pauper'. Under the 1890 Lunacy Act, it became permissible to detain a mentally disordered person for up to three days.

Police and Criminal Evidence Act 1984

If the place of safety is a police station, the safeguards of the Police and Criminal Evidence Act 1984 (PACE) will apply, and an appropriate adult will have to be summoned [Code C, para 1.4] as well as an ASW, although it is unclear as to what the former will do that the ASW cannot.

Warrant to search for and remove a patient under s.135

An Approved Social Worker can apply on oath to a magistrate for a warrant authorising a police officer to enter private premises, if necessary using force. An application can be made

> ... if there is reasonable cause to suspect that a person believed to be suffering from a mental disorder (a) has been, or is being ill-treated, neglected or kept otherwise than under proper control in any jurisdiction of the justice, or (b) being unable to care for himself, is living alone ... .

(Mental Health Act 1983, s.135)

The person may be removed to a place of safety for a period not exceeding 72 hours, starting with the time the person arrives at the place of safety, so that consideration may be given to making an application for compulsory detention under the 1983 Mental Health Act (MHA), or for alternative arrangements to be made for their care and treatment. The application must be in writing and placed before a magistrate. In an emergency, the magistrate may be approached at home.

Although a hospital is the preferred place of safety, in reality it is often a police station even though this is contrary to the advice in the Code of Practice.

Admission through the courts (part III)

Persons may be admitted to hospital from the Crown Court as a result of criminal proceedings. This can be as a result of pleading that their mental state makes it impossible for them to have a fair trial. The trial may still go on and the jury can still order the person to be detained in a psychiatric hospital, usually a medium secure unit, although this will depend upon the nature and extent of the offending behaviour (Criminal Procedure (Insanity and Unfitness to Plead) Act, 1991).

As a social worker you could have had prior involvement with them and/or their families and be asked to provide social circumstance reports. You may need to respond to the family's need for information and assistance whilst the patient is detained. Most areas also operate projects like 'Diversion from Custody' which are aimed at keeping people who are minor offenders but have mental health problems out of the court system. This work will involve social workers, nurses and police officers working together.

Part III of the 1983 Mental Health Act

Part III of the 1983 Mental Health Act (MHA) deals with patients involved in criminal proceedings or under sentence. Except for s.35, before using their powers under Part III, the court requires two medical recommendations (one from a s.12 approved doctor). Written medical reports are normally sent to court in advance of the hearing and doctors should be prepared to give oral evidence if requested. The main sections of Part III are as follows:

- Section 35   Remand to hospital for report.

- Section 36   Remand to hospital for treatment.

- Section 37   Hospital order.

- Section 38   Interim hospital orders.

- Section 41   Restriction order.

- Sections 47–53   Transfer of prisoners to hospital.

- Section 45A   Power to direct hospital admission.

Home Office Mental Health Unit

The Mental Health Unit was formerly known as C3 Division and it exercises the Home Secretary's powers in respect of restricted patients under the 1983 MHA. A restriction order is made by a Crown Court when it is necessary to protect the public from serious harm. The effect of a restriction order is that the Home Secretary's permission is required before a restricted patient can be discharged from hospital, transferred or given leave of absence. A Mental Health Review Tribunal (MHRT) can also discharge a restricted patient.

The Home Secretary's main statutory functions in respect of restricted patients include:

- consenting to or directing their discharge (with conditions if necessary);

- consenting to leave of absence;

- consenting to a transfer;

- recalling a conditionally discharged patient to hospital;

- providing statements to MHRTs; and

- considering reports prepared on behalf of restricted and conditionally discharged patients. Social workers (including ASWs) may be asked to produce these reports.

CASE STUDY

Following James Hadfield's attempted assassination of King George III in the nineteenth century, the courts were concerned that he might provide a risk to others in the future. Parliament passed the Safe Custody of Insane Persons Charged with Offences Act (1800), which was the forerunner of the current restriction order. The Royal Commission on the Law Relating to Mental Illness and Mental Deficiency (1957) recommended the current restriction order. The Committee felt that the Home Secretary was the logical choice as the pivotal authority for this role.

Human rights and the admission process

Brammer (2003) offers a clear view of the relationship between the European Human Rights legislation and the operation of the 1983 MHA. In particular Article 5 provides the right not to be deprived of liberty except in specific cases, which includes being of unsound mind. Through adjudications in a number of cases the following minimum principles have been determined:

- detention must follow a legally prescribed procedure;

- a medical assessment of the person's mental health must be obtained;

- the disorder must be of an extent to justify compulsory admission; and

- continued detention can only occur if the mental disorder continues.

(Brammer, p.345)

Under present legislation the rights of patients who are detained under a section of the MHA are protected through various aspects of the Code of Practice and sections of the MHA itself. These are too many to go through thoroughly but the main ones that you may be involved in are: treatment; application to Hospital Managers' Review and Application to the Mental Health Review Tribunal.

Detention in hospital

As a social worker you need to understand what happens to patients when they are detained in hospital, what to advise their carers and what they should expect from the hospital and community services.

Information for detained patients

Patients detained under the 1983 Mental Health Act (MHA) and their nearest relative (NR) have the right to certain information which must be provided by the hospital managers after admission. Hospital managers must ensure that the patient receives information, where relevant, in respect of the:

- powers of the hospital managers, NR and RMO to discharge a patient from their detention;

- availability of free specialist mental health legal representation;

- legal position in relation to consent to treatment under MHA Part IV;

- existence of the Code of Practice to guide care health and social care professionals in the performance of their duties;

- role and function of the Mental Health Act Commission (MHAC);

- rules relating to the sending and receipt of mail under s.134 (in high security hospitals).

The hospital managers *must* identify a suitable member of staff e.g. an experienced nurse or doctor to give the required information to a detained patient. Information should be given orally to the patient and in writing. Rights information leaflets are produced by the Department of Health (and Welsh Office) to enable Hospital Managers to comply with s.132 of the MHA.

Informal patients and those subject to Guardianship under s.7 do not enjoy a similar entitlement although, as a matter of good practice, they should be informed of their legal status and rights.

Without information the patient and their advocates are at a disadvantage should they wish to challenge detention or refuse treatment. This may mean several attempts have to be made before satisfactory understanding is achieved. The MHAC on their visits to hospitals and social services will check that this has been properly recorded and ask patients about the information that they have received.

Treatment in hospital

Medical treatment means a range of interventions including drug treatments, nursing care, therapeutic interventions, and could include behaviour modification and task-centred work. Where medical treatment is given it should only be for the mental disorder that the patient is suffering. This provides a degree of safeguard for the patients but is open to interpretation and professional discretion. When a patient's life is under threat the situation is far more complex. Where to draw the line between physical and mental disorder is usually a matter for professional decision-making and rulings through the courts.

ACTIVITY **3.4**

Why is it important for patients to obtain information? How do you know that they understand the information? Who checks?

Medication

One of the most important innovations in the 1983 Mental Health Act (MHA) was the regulation of treatment for mental disorder for non-consenting patients detained under Part IV of the 1983 MHA. The medical treatment of informal patients in psychiatric hospitals in many ways mirrors that of patients in general hospitals and they have the right to refuse treatment as well as discharge themselves without conditions (subject to s.5 holding powers). As the vast majority of patients are informal the common law applies to their treatment for mental disorder in the same way as any other health problem.

Consent is the voluntary and continuing permission of the patient to receive a particular treatment, based on an adequate knowledge of the purpose, nature, likely effects and risks of that treatment, including the likelihood of its success and any alternatives to it. Permission given under any unfair or undue pressure is not 'consent' (Code of Practice, para 15.13). This exception is based on the assumption that a person with mental disorder may have impaired judgement as a consequence of their illness and therefore may be declining treatment that if they were a little better they would accept. This is an uncomfortable position to be in and it can put social workers in the invidious position of trying to work with service users in an empowering way whilst being a member of a multi-disciplinary team giving invasive treatment against the person's wishes.

Elsewhere the ranges of medical interventions are discussed (Chapter 2) and it is worth reflecting that prescribed drugs for the treatment of mental disorder account for around 25% of all prescriptions issued through the NHS (Bartlett and Sandland 2003, p.326). The treatment of chronic disorders like schizophrenia alone is estimated to cost over £1 billion. Even with this huge spend patients report varying degrees of satisfaction with these medications and the relapse rate continues to be at a level that stretches service level provision and the side effects cause some distress to many users.

Electroconvulsive therapy (ECT)

Electroconvulsive therapy (ECT) is a form of somatic treatment for certain psychiatric conditions in which an electrical current is applied to the brain through two electrodes placed on the skull. ECT was developed in the 1930s when it was believed that epilepsy and schizophrenia were mutually exclusive although the use of convulsive therapy can be traced back to the use of the Mediterranean torpedo fish which produces a relatively small electric shock and was placed across the patient's brow (Eldergill, 1997). The present technique has been modified over the years. A consultant anaesthetist administers the pre-medication and anaesthetic and a psychiatrist administers the ECT. Experienced psychiatric nurses are present to support the patient. Most patients suffer some short-term memory loss for up to one to two months post-ECT. The National Institute of Clinical Excellence (NICE) has endorsed the value of ECT as an accepted part of modern psychiatric treatment (April 2003). As from 2003 the Royal College of Psychiatrists (RCOP) recommends that all administration of ECT should comply with the new standards and safeguards set by ECTAS (ECT accreditation service). ECT clinics approved by ECTAS will in future be identified on the RCOP website.

Emergency treatment

This is provided under s. 62 and is limited to the minimum treatment necessary to respond to the emergency. This may not always be dramatic life-saving situations but could be for 'lesser emergencies'. Evidence suggests that from time to time this section has been used to include patients who are in hospital informally and presenting difficult behaviour on the hospital wards (Bartlett and Sandham, 2003, p.390).

Restraint and seclusion

Restraint may be necessary from time to time and should only be carried out by trained staff who are able to exercise minimal force that is consistent with resolution of the behaviour. The use of restraint is controversial and dates back to the use of straightjackets and other mechanical restraints. In the present time investigations and inquiries have thrown doubt upon the capabilities of some staff (MHAC, 2001, para 4.49).

The Code of Practice defines seclusion as 'the supervised confinement of a patient in a room, which may be locked to protect others from significant harm (para 19.16). However in a recent case the Court of Appeal used an alternative definition, which may be wider and therefore may cover other forms of intervention than this definition covers (the case of R on the application of Colonel Munjaz v Mersey Care NHS Trust; S v Airedale NHS Trust (2003) EWCA Civ 1036). The appeal court also said that the Code should be observed by all hospitals unless they have a good reason for departing from it in relation to an individual patient or a group of patients sharing similar characteristics. Failure to follow the Code of Practise may expose the secluder to a legal challenge.

CASE STUDY

David Bennett died in a medium secure unit having been restrained for 25 minutes follow-ing an incident in which racial abuse was levelled at him. This incident contributed to his death. There appeared not to be a doctor present and the nurse gave him medication. This was outside their legal authority which even in an emergency does not permit a nurse to authorise medication to be administered without the patient's consent. The Inquiry also raised important concerns about racist practices in the NHS (Bennett Inquiry, 2004).

1983 MHA Code of Practice

In the same case, the Court *concluded that the Code should be observed by all hospitals unless they have a good reason for departing from it in relation to an individual patient.* Therefore seclusion should always comply with the guidance in the MHA Code of Practice, 19.16 – 19.23 (March 1999 edition). A copy of the Code should be available on the ward for anyone to inspect.

Leaving hospital

Discharge

Most patients in psychiatric hospitals are informal patients and they can discharge them-selves when they wish (subject to the holding powers of s.5 of the MHA). In practice patients will discuss discharge with their RMO and others once they begin to feel better; this may be when medication has begun to work or when circumstances at home or in the community would allow them to leave hospital. This may necessitate social workers becoming involved in order to identify support services and systems that could be avail-able for the patient and their families.

Where discharge by the patient is not possible the 1983 MHA provides two channels of appeal against detention in hospital, [i] to the hospital managers and to [ii] a Mental Health Review Tribunal whereby the continued detention of the patient can be challenged and it is to these that we now turn. Continued justification for detention can only be con-sidered if it is a proportionate response to the perceived risks that might occur should the patient be discharged (case of H *v* Mental Health Review Tribunal, North and North East London Region, 2001).

Hospital Managers' Review

Compulsory detention under the 1983 Mental Health Act is not merely a medical matter. It also raises important issues relating to the civil liberty of the individual concerned. Since it is the hospital managers who are the formal detaining authority under the MHA, the Act permits a patient to request a review of their detention. This varies according to the estab-lishment concerned. In an NHS Trust Hospital or Special Health Authority it is those responsible for the administration of the hospital and in an Independent Hospital it is the registered person under the Care Standards Act 2000. It is important to distinguish hospi-tal managers from other staff who may also be referred to as managers, e.g. a directorate manager or patients' services manager is not a hospital manager under the MHA. The 1983 MHA Code of Practice recommends that hospital managers consider holding a review, if the patient requests it; or if detention is renewed under s.20; or if the RMO issues a barring order (s.25) opposing a nearest relative's request for discharge of the patient.

Mental Health Review Tribunal

In certain circumstances an individual subject to the 1983 MHA or their nearest relative (NR) may appeal to a Mental Health Review Tribunal (MHRT). The relevant legislation may be found in Part V of the MHA and the MHRT Rules. There are also rights of appeal for individuals who are received into guardianship (s.7) or subject to supervised discharge (s.25(A)). Patients who are detained under a short-term power with a maximum duration of 72 hours or less cannot appeal to a MHRT (i.e. s.4, s.5(2), s.5(4), s.135 and s.136).

The purpose of the MHRT is to hear the patient's appeal against detention and reception into guardianship or supervised discharge. The hospital managers (NHS Trust or Independent Hospital registered to take detained patients) or if subject to guardianship, the Local Social Services Department (LSSD) must justify the need for the continued use of the Act. The Act sets out the circumstances in which a MHRT can discharge a detained patient. The Tribunal also has additional powers to recommend: leave of absence; transfer to another hospital; delayed discharge; supervised discharge and guardianship.

A legal member sits with a consultant psychiatrist and a lay member. All members are appointed by the Lord Chancellor's Office. Each panel member considers the case on its individual merits. A MHRT is a court and as such a legal member always chairs proceedings. This person is referred to as The President of the Tribunal.

Always remind the patient that they are entitled to be represented by a solicitor with specialist mental health experience, absolutely free of charge under the legal aid scheme. This is especially important as the patient/NR may be worried about paying the fee. The solicitor may decide to involve an expert witness, e.g. independent psychiatrist, social worker or psychologist.

In all cases a social work report will be required and these can be compiled by a social worker who need not be an ASW. There has been some concern about the quality of some social work reports. This report should cover the circumstances surrounding the admission and importantly the situation at present. This should include the patient's financial circumstance, accommodation, opportunities for employment, family and other support systems and a commentary upon the available social service support and supervised discharge into the community. Eldergill (1998) provides excellent guidance in this area.

ACTIVITY **3.5**

You arrive at the hospital ward to meet your patient with whom you have already established a professional relationship. She was admitted two days ago and this is your first visit to the ward. She tells you that the staff have said that as she is detained on a s.2 she can apply for either a Hospital Managers' Review or a Tribunal. She wants to know which one is best. What is your advice?

It is worth reminding detained patients (and their NR) that under s.2, s.3 and s.37 they can request *both* a Managers' Review and a Mental Health Review Tribunal.

Court of Protection

Part VII of the 1983 Mental Health Act (MHA) aims to protect the property and financial affairs of an individual (referred to in the MHA as a patient) who is incapable of acting for themselves because of a mental disorder. Mental disorder is widely defined and may include people with learning disabilities, mental illness or a brain injury. The MHA also provides safeguards for anyone authorised by the Court of Protection (Court) to manage the patient's finances (referred to in the MHA as a receiver).

The administrative work of the Court of Protection is carried out by the Public Guardianship Office (PGO). The PGO is an Executive Agency within the Lord Chancellor's Department. It offers advice and information as well as support. The Court is headed by the Master of the Court of Protection and based in London.

RESEARCH SUMMARY

Prior to the 1959 MHA it was presumed that all patients formally detained in hospital under the MHA were unable to manage their financial affairs. The Royal Commission on the Law Relating to Mental Illness and Mental Deficiency (Percy Commission, 1957) concluded that a person's legal status could not in itself indicate whether they were capable of handling their own financial affairs. It recommended that each person's circumstances should be decided on the basis of an objective test of capacity (although there is no actual test in existence).

Treatment in the community

The Care Programme Approach (CPA)

The CPA is a major part of the government's mental health policy. In September 1990 the Department of Health issued guidance (HC (90) LASSL (90) 11) introducing this approach that would provide a network of care in the community for service users who experience severe mental disorder. One aim was to minimise the risk of patients losing contact with services. Another was to meet the needs of the service user and provide a degree of co-ordination that would reduce the risk to the community of the small number of people who have mental disorder and a history of dangerousness or violent behaviour. It is more than an aftercare arrangement and should provide a framework for innovative and assertive care.

The CPA applies to all service users aged 16 or over and under the care of specialist mental health services and involves the following:

- A systematic assessment of the health and social care needs of the service user.

- A care plan which has been agreed by all concerned including wherever possible the service user, GP, social worker, carer, CPN and other members of the multi disciplinary team.

- The nomination of a key worker who takes the responsibility to co-ordinate care and to keep in close contact with the service user.

- The whole plan is to be reviewed regularly (six monthly) to determine the progress towards the service user's goals and to make changes to the plan where necessary.

This is usually organised around a two level approach, namely Standard for those who require a minimal service and Enhanced which caters for service users who have long-term and severe mental disorder that cause significant social dysfunction. This latter category could include those who are assessed to be at risk of suicide, self-harm or neglect.

It is the duty of the health and social services under the 1983 MHA s.117 to provide after-care for patients who have been detained in hospital for treatment or who are subject to guardianship. This is a duty that is imposed on the statutory services and will involve social workers and other professionals who could act as a key worker overseeing the operation of the plan. This is a part of the Care Programme Approach and will involve a risk assessment. The plan comes to a conclusion when the services decide in consultation with the service user that the service user's needs have changed. The service user is under no obligation to accept after-care although in reality this may mean a delay in the discharge from hospital (Brammer, 2003, p.356).

What do social workers do?

As a social worker you may become the key worker who will be responsible for among other things:

- contributing to care assessment and planning;

- monitoring and reviewing the care plan;

- being familiar with the service user's circumstances;

- maintaining close therapeutic contact with the service user;

- contributing to, attending and possibly chairing the review;

- ensuring that the service user is empowered;

- monitoring the services that are delivered and promoting culturally appropriate services.

Community Mental Health Trusts and community based teams provide the cornerstone of present day services and in some areas include assertive outreach teams and 24-hour services while others have none whatsoever. No matter what services are on offer it is clearly the government's intention that nurses, medical practitioners and social workers should work together to provide better services for service users. Recent research by Carpenter et al. (2003) suggests that in the move towards integration social workers are finding it most difficult to adapt and are among the most stressed of the professional groups.

ACTIVITY **3.6**

Why are social workers finding it difficult to work with other professions? Write down three possible reasons and compare with the notes below. Justify your reasons.

You may have come up with a variety of suggestions including the following:

- Social workers are typically the only professional people who are not from a medical background.

- Social workers assess the service user in their social context and may develop a view that social factors affect the service user's mental health and that service users may be victims.

- Social workers do not have as clear a role as other workers and consequently cannot draw upon the same professional guidelines as nurses and doctors.

- Social workers, unlike nurses, have not trained under doctors and are more likely to challenge their opinions.

- Uniquely social work is embedded in the ideas of social exclusion and oppression.

Supervised discharge (s.25A)

The Mental Health (Patients in the Community) Act 1995 is commonly referred to as supervised discharge under s.25A. The purpose of supervised discharge is to ensure that a person who has been detained in hospital for treatment receives after-care services under s.117 of the 1983 Mental Health Act. Supervised discharge applies to people over 16 who are currently detained under s.3 (admission for treatment), s.37 (hospital order imposed by the courts) or s.47 or s.48 (transfer of prisoners to hospital). Supervised discharge initially lasts for six months and can be renewed for a further six months and then for one year at a time. Supervised discharge requires the patient to live in a particular place, attend a particular place at set times for treatment, occupation, education or training; and allow the supervisor or someone authorised by them, access to the home. A MHRT may recommend that an application for supervised discharge be considered by the patient's RMO.

Guardianship (s.7)

The purpose of guardianship is to enable patients to receive community care where it cannot be provided without the use of compulsory powers. It establishes an authoritative framework for working with the patient and must form part of their overall care and treatment plan. A guardianship application can be made in respect of anyone aged 16 or over who meets the statutory criteria. Patients detained under the 1983 Mental Health Act, informal patients and individuals brought before the courts can all be considered for guardianship. In addition, a Mental Health Review Tribunal (MHRT) can recommend a patient be considered for guardianship. A guardian's powers under the Act may be described as *essential powers* as they only authorise restricting the patient's liberty in the three essential ways described in s.8. This confers on the responsible local social services authority – RLSSA (s.34 (3)) – or the person named as guardian, the power to require the patient to [i] reside at a specified place; [ii] attend at specific places and at set times for medical treatment, occupation, education or training; [iii] allow access at any place where s/he resides, to any registered medical practitioner, Approved Social Worker (ASW) or other specified person. The guardian has no power over the patient's finances or property and cannot consent to treatment on the patient's behalf. Guardianship lasts for up to six months from the date it was accepted. It can be renewed for a further six months and thereafter at yearly intervals. Guardianship may remain in force if the person is admitted to hospital as an informal patient or for assessment under s.2 or s.4.

Future mental health legislation

When I wrote the first edition of this book there was fever in the air with the excitement not to mention controversy over the imminent arrival of new legislation. After eight years of negotiations, prevarication, amendments government ministers decided on 23 March 2006 to abandon their plans to introduce new mental health legislation at least for the foreseeable future. This was much to the delight of those who were very concerned about issues like compulsory treatment in the community and the detention of people who were believed to be mentally ill and posed a risk to them or to the community. However these aspects are likely to be included in the new bill that will amend the 1983 Mental Health Act.

This new legislation will be shorter and more streamlined and will effectively amend the existing legislation. The government's aim is that these changes will reflect the impact of service modernisation and will be easier for service users and professional to understand. The former is easier to see how this will occur but the latter seem to be very remote as the bill will add to rather than replace the present legislation. It is in the other objectives to promote patients' safeguards and to protect patients and the public from harm that we see the real reasons that have driven the government to this point.

To get at the underlying reasons behind this legislation it is necessary to take a short trip back to July 1996 when Dr Lin Russell and her two young daughters were the victims of a frenzied attack in a country lane in Chillenden near Canterbury, Kent. Mother and elder daughter were bludgeoned to death, the younger daughter 9-year old Josie somehow survived. A year after this attack Michael Stone was arrested but persistently denied that this crime was carried out by him and in fact his later confession was one that was shouted through the prison cell wall where he had been remanded. Police built up a picture of what happened, based partly on Josie's recollections, although she couldn't identify Stone and partly on the confessions to a cellmate. He also has a record for serious violence, including a hammer attack but in quite dissimilar circumstances.

The mental health authorities knew Michael Stone in 1994 when he had been compulsorily admitted to the then De La Pole Hospital in Hull but doctors there decided that his condition was untreatable and he was discharged into the community. Stone was diagnosed as having a psychopathic personality and there is conflicting evidence about how dangerous professionals thought he was, even though this was shortly before he murdered Lin and Megan Russell. By all accounts he was a rather pathetic person with a long-standing history of multiple drug misuse something which he readily admits but he is adamant that what he suffers with is drug induced psychosis not severe personality disorder. Could his behaviour have been predicted? What could have been done to better protect the public? Was he bad not mad? Would it be good law to change the legislation to respond to the minority of people like Stone? Answers to these questions raise considerable issues about liberty, mental health and protection of the public.

To their credit the *Independent on Sunday* have been at the forefront of a campaign to get the government to drop the Mental Health Bill arguing successfully as it turns out that the Bill was an inappropriate response to what is in reality a statistically rare event. In fact the biggest threat that mental health patients pose is to themselves not to others and that you are twenty times more likely to be killed by a sane person than by a mental health patient. David Hewitt in a visionary article in November 2005 suggests that the 1983 Act had been modified so much over the last 20 years that sweeping change was in any case now unnecessary (Hewitt, November 2005).

Meanwhile Michael Stone through his legal representatives is fighting to keep from publication an independent report by Robert Francis QC which has so far been repressed for over six years. This report it is claimed describes in detail the multiple failures of the 'system' that should have been more alert and responsive to the widely held view that Stone was a very dangerous man who had expressed ideas about hurting people before he committed this latest crime. Stone is objecting because of the disclosure of his private life. Of course Shaun Russell and his daughter Josie are arguing that the report must be published in order that agencies can learn the lessons and to prevent similar attacks.

The situation is that many people who are considered to be 'anti-social' and even described as psychopaths are often well known to services but do not as a rule commit serious crimes and it was impossible to predict those who were a real threat to the public. This of course poses a big problem for future legislation since the assessment of severe personality disorder is difficult and such conditions in any event are very resistant to treatment.

There will need to be considerable skill exercised if the government's objectives are to be met and the rights of patients and citizens preserved. To err too much on the side of caution could result in mental hospitals becoming like another form of prison full of people with so-called personality disorder, which by its very nature could be considered untreatable. An over zealous response may also result in the Michael Stones of the world, keeping well away from services for fear of being subject to compulsory treatment

On 23 March 2006 the Health Minister, Rosie Winterton, announced fresh proposals for a Bill to amend the existing 1983 Mental Health Act. This new Bill will be much shorter than the now discarded Mental Health Bill of 2004 and will introduce supervised treatment in the community to ensure treatment compliance for those who were on a compulsory detention order and have been discharged into the community. This is designed to protect both patients and to improve public safety.

At the same time mental disorder will be redefined to make it simpler and to remove the treatability condition. These changes are also to provide treatment for patients who are in need to prevent them harming themselves or others.

The new Bill, which will be introduced when Parliamentary time allows, will:

- *Introduce supervised treatment in the community for suitable patients following an initial period of detention and treatment in hospital. This will help ensure that patients continue to comply with treatment and enable action to be taken to prevent their relapsing in the community. The introduction of treatment in the community reflects modern service provision enabling patients to be treated according to their individual needs and circumstances.*

- *Expand the skill base of professionals who are responsible for the treatment of patients treated without their consent.*

- *Improve patient safeguards by taking order-making powers with regard to the Mental Health Review Tribunal. We are currently considering across government the precise terms of the changes, and will continue to consult with stakeholders.*

- *Reflect a widespread consensus and the views of the Joint Committee and will introduce a new, simplified single definition of mental disorder to ensure that people who require treatment to prevent harm to themselves or others are able to receive it.*

- *Replace the 'treatability test' (which currently results in some people with personality disorder being inappropriately excluded from the treatment they need), keep, as recommended by the Joint Committee, the exclusion for drug and alcohol dependency, and preserve the effect of the Act as it relates to people with learning disabilities.*

- *Amend the current Act to remedy an ECHR incompatibility in relation to the Nearest Relative. At the same time, we will bring the Act into line with the Civil Partnership Act 2004 in relation to the Nearest Relative provisions.*

The Bill will be used as the vehicle for introducing the Bournewood safeguards, through amending the Mental Capacity Act 2005. These safeguards are for people who lack capacity and are deprived of their liberty but do not receive mental health legislation safeguards.

We will address safeguards for children treated on the basis of parental consent through the Children Act 1989. Children detained under the Mental Health Act will continue to receive the same safeguards as adults.

We will also look at ways that we can continue to pursue other patient safeguards, such as advocacy, through other means. (Press release DoH, 23 March 2006)

Mental Capacity Act 2005

The Mental Capacity Act received Royal Assent in April 2005 and after a period of consultation about the detail of implementation will come into force in April 2007. This legislation has been a long time in the making, can be traced back to the Law Commission in 1989 and has undergone a number of revisions before the present statute. This Act governs decision-making for those in society who have lost or expect to lose the capacity to make independent decisions. It covers virtually all aspects of living including personal and financial matters.

It is expected that once the Act is implemented social care professionals will play a crucial and at times pivotal role for people who are lacking in capacity and being cared for by a range of people including professionals. This Act brings about a test of capacity thereby removing the possibility of someone being labelled as incapable solely because of a particular diagnosis. The assumption will be that the person has capacity to make decisions unless proven otherwise. For instance a person with a diagnosis of learning disability or dementia will, irrespective of this condition, still be assumed to be capable of decision.

Making an unwise decision is of itself not enough to assume that the person lacks the capacity to make other decisions. Any decisions made on behalf of adults who lack capacity must be made in line with their rights and freedoms and must be the least restricted option.

Social Care professionals may be involved in:

- Protecting vulnerable people from exploitation or abuse.

- Providing information to service users which will require in many cases considerable communication skills.

- Using the services of specialist staff where communication difficulties exceed the conventional skill set of social work or social care staff.

- Support the family or carers to help them to understand and recognise that the service user can make their own decisions.

- Assessing the service user so as to provide information of the social functioning of the service user.

- Play a key part in providing what is in the best interests of the person being cared for.

(Adapted from Making Decisions: leaflet 3 Helping people who have difficulty in making decisions for themselves available as a free download on www.dca.gov.uk?consult/family/leaf3.htm)

CHAPTER SUMMARY

The area of mental health law is a complex one and this chapter has introduced you to some of the provisions and responsibilities placed on the various people who may make decisions about people who are extremely vulnerable. Although much of this chapter has focused on the Approved Social Worker and the responsibilities that they currently have, it is absolutely essential that all mental health and generic social workers have a basic understanding of the 1983 Mental Health Act, MHA Code of Practice, Memorandum on Parts I to VI, VII and X of the MHA and the successor legislation.

A new law was introduced in 2004 in Scotland with increased emphasis upon a social welfare model of mental health. In Wales the Assembly is setting out its vision for improving and modernising mental health services.

FURTHER READING

There are numerous texts that you will find helpful and often it is a matter of preference as to which one you will want to use.

Christopher Curran and Catherine Grimshaw are well respected for considering a number of aspects of the 1983 Mental Health Act as well the use of seclusion and the role of the Approved Social Worker. Their articles have regularly appeared in the *OpenMind Journal*. *OpenMind* is a service user/practitioner journal and is well worth subscribing to. In addition, they have published a number of other articles on mental health law, policy and practice in *Medicine, Science and the Law*; *Psychiatric Bulletin* and *Psychiatric Care* (see bibliography for details).

Richard Jones' *Mental Health Act Manual*, 2002, has become the most used text in this area and although it is specifically focused upon the interpretation of the Mental Health Act 1983 it also covers the Mental Health Act 1983 Code of Practice, Mental Health Act 1983 Memorandum on Parts I to VI, VIII and X and Guidance Notes published by the Mental Health Act Commission

Bartlett and Sandland (2nd ed) have produced an informative text (2003) about mental health law policy and practice that will provide some of the missing detail to this chapter.

Professor Anselm Eldergill's *Mental Health Law Review Tribunals: Law and Practice* (1998) is a standard mental health law text book. It provides an excellent reference text for solicitors, social workers and mental health professionals on Mental Health Review Tribunals and many other matters.

Chapter 4

Working with vulnerable people: mental health in children and adolescents

There is always one moment in childhood when the door opens and lets the future in.
Graham Greene (1940)

Introduction

In this chapter you will consider the kind of issues and knowledge that social workers need in order to carry out effective work with children and adolescents who have poor mental health. This will help you to understand the nature of these mental health problems and disorders and how to respond to them. Later on the focus is on working with adolescents who are dealing with the problems of eating disorders, self-harm, dissociative disorder and depression.

The government undertook a crucial policy initative under the general heading of Every Child Matters, which will transform children's services, The Children Act 2004 provides the legal framework for improving children's lives. The government state that it 'is to encourage integrated planning, commissioning and delivery of services as well as improve the coordination of individual and joint inspections in local authorites. The legislation is enabling rather than prescriptive and provides local authoriteis with a considerable amount of flexibility in the way they implement its provisions'. (www.dfes.gov.uk)

What social workers need to know to work effectively with children and adolescents

Social work with children and adolescents has until recently received little attention. However the government has endorsed the need for community and specialist services for this important group. Social workers have the skills necessary to work effectively with adolescents and to be key workers in multi-disciplinary settings.

There are many approaches that social workers and others use, some more effective than others. All have behind them a set of assumptions that raise issues for you, the service user and their carers. For example when working with an adolescent who displays behaviour associated with depression is the adolescent the primary client or is it the worried parent? Working with the adolescent to help them to articulate their needs may be at odds with what their family want and believe should happen. A child may be bottling up feelings because they inwardly feel that to open up is to risk alienation of the family, yet it may be in their interests to express these feelings.

As a social worker you need to understand what the various mental disorders are in order that you can work alongside other professionals as well as undertaking direct work yourself. This is a complex area and you need to resist making simplistic assessments of complex situations and playing the role of amateur psychiatrist. Where your strengths lie is in using an empowering approach when you can work with people to help them discover explanations that they understand and ways of intervening that actually work for them. The real experts are the service users who have experienced for themselves the impact of mental disorder.

You could be working with children, adolescents and families as part of a team or approach or in your own right. The kind of problems that you could be working with can be categorised as follows:

Under -5s

- communication problems;
- sleeping difficulties;
- unusually strong or long-lasting tantrums;
- children who are suffering anxieties after major trauma or major life events such as divorce or separation of parents.

School-age but pre-adolescent children

- hyperactive problems;
- bed-wetting or soiling;
- relationship problems;
- behavioural problems at home or school;
- school refusal problems.

Adolescents

- eating disorders;
- behavioural problems;
- anxiety states;
- self-harm;
- depression;
- substance abuse.

Of course before social workers get involved these problems and disorders must be perceived as either dysfunctional or disruptive and therefore it is essential to determine if this behaviour is within 'normal' or acceptable limits. Being in a position to do this requires that you have an understanding of the usual progression of children and adolescents and some knowledge of the kind of mental health problems and mental disorder that young people face. There are some disorders that are more closely associated with children and adolescents, even though they may also occur in adults.

Definitions of mental health in the context of adolescent development

Chapter 2 covered the main elements that make up a diagnosis of mental disorder and help us to appreciate mental health problems. It is worth revisiting this in the context of children and adolescents as there is a view held by many people that what we see as mental health problems are, in effect, simply signs of growing up that all of us have experience of. In other words if these problems are normal for adolescents the chances are that the young people will grow out of them and therefore we should intervene only as a last resort. The other view is that we should intervene earlier with relatively minor mental health problems to try to arrest them before they develop into something more serious. As a social worker you need to be clear about where you stand in this respect, as much of our work is at the cross-over point between these views.

Adolescence is a period of development in our lives that is characterised by massive learning and assimilation of ideas as well as having to become a social being learning all the social mores. Writing about adolescence and the life course Crawford and Walker suggest that:

> … *it is the critical process of the development of self, the search for identity and the development of relationships, for example with friends, and the changing nature of relationships, for example with families, that are a central feature of this period of an individual's life.*
>
> (Crawford and Walker, 2003, p.70)

It can be an intense time with significant pressures put on young people to perform at school and college and to reach developmental milestones. For some it can be the lack of opportunity and the disinterest of others in them that causes feelings of social exclusion and isolation. At the same time these pressures can produce stress, which as we have seen is one of the key intervening variables in the probable cause of mental health problems and onset of disorder (Chapter 2 provides more detail).

This needs to be put alongside on the one hand the popular view, often seen in the media, that adolescents are becoming more and more troublesome, whilst on the other hand is the romantic view of childhood innocence. Of course neither of these views is totally accurate and they illustrate the ambivalent attitude often shown by adults and the community at large towards adolescents.

RESEARCH SUMMARY

In 1999 the ONS carried out the first nationally representative survey of the mental health of children and adolescents. Results indicate that there are inequalities in children's mental health depending on their household's income. Children from households with lower gross weekly incomes were more likely than those from households with higher incomes to display a mental disorder of some kind. For most income brackets, children aged 11 to 15 were more likely to have a mental disorder than those aged 5 to 10. In addition, children were more likely to suffer from poor mental health if their parents were unemployed, and if their parents had few or no educational qualifications.

Prevalence of mental disorders among children: by gross weekly household income and age of child, 1999: Social Trends, 31

Mental health problems and disorders in children and adolescents

One of the challenges to us is to understand the nature and extent of mental health problems and mental disorder that children and adolescents experience. The Health Advisory

Service (1995) estimated that of the children and adolescent population in the UK the following will at some point experience mental health problems and disorders as below:

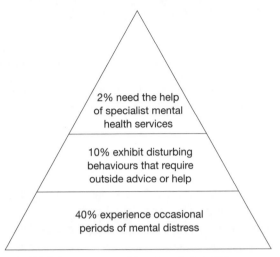

Figure 4.1: *Children and Adolescent use of Services in the UK*

These UK statistics can be compared with a 1999 study in the USA that showed that almost 21% of US children and adolescents aged between 9 and 17 had a diagnosable mental health or addictive problem and that for the more serious mental disorder the figure was 11%. The World Health Organisation predicts that there will be a significant increase in psychiatric disorders among children and adolescents that will place such disorders as one of the five most serious causes of death and disability among children (National Institute of Mental Health, 2003).

Good mental health is more than the absence of mental illness and the Mental Health Foundation (1999) suggested that mentally healthy children and adolescents will be those who can:

- develop psychologically, emotionally, creatively, intellectually and physically;
- sustain mutually satisfying relationships with others;
- use and enjoy solitude;
- become aware of others and empathise with them;
- play and learn;
- develop a sense of right and wrong;
- deal with problems and setbacks from time to time.

These development indicators are important for you to understand as they set the context within which you will develop your practice as a social worker, but of course they also require interpretation and reference to any previous history of mental health problems before considering someone's mental health. Equally valid is to get the young person's view of their mental health.

Think back to your childhood and adolescence and using the above list see how well you managed to meet these developmental goals. How many of the above proved at some time in your development to be problematic? What constitutes 'normal' difficulties and what constitutes development that is not normal? Who is it that decides about this? Is it possible that you met the entire list but still had mental health problems?

Of course different people will have had different experiences and some of those will be determined by your gender, ethnicity, family circumstances and, structural reasons like poverty.

Some young people who have experienced mental health problems and disorder believe that these lists do not cover all that is necessary for positive mental health.

Don't lose sight of the reality that it is adults who have determined what is satisfactory or not satisfactory about child and adolescent mental health. Walker points out that there is little evidence of young people having been consulted about their mental health problems. Consequently it is possible that what adults may want from children may well be at odds with what the young people wish for themselves. (Walker, 2003)

Common mental health disorders

Although mental disorder can affect people of all ages there are some aspects that are more usually associated with certain age groups. Some of the more common mental disorders and mental health problems for adolescents are set out below.

Depressive disorders

These include major depression, bipolar and adjustment disorder that adversely affect the mood, energy and general social functioning of the young person. Most adolescents from time to time suffer from mood swings, depression and periods of hyperactivity, but the presence of these depressive disorders is distinguished from these by the duration of the symptoms and the extent that it interferes with everyday life.

There is a growing belief that a small minority of young people show signs of depressive disorders much earlier than has previously been thought and that this may occur during childhood. Depression often affects males and females differently but with both it is often difficult to uncover whether they are unhappy or depressed. The line between this unhappiness, which is short-term, and the longer-term nature of depression is quite difficult to draw. Learning how to do this is down to experience and recognising some of the key signs.

The points at which concerns are raised relate to the extent of the behaviours and their intensity. For instance going into your bedroom for short periods and playing loud music is all part of being an adolescent, but going into your room, locking the door and refusing to have meals or to talk with the family is a point of concern if this lasts more than a few hours. This is a matter of degree and intensity and needs to be compared with previous behaviours.

Depressive disorders are closely associated with an increased risk of suicidal behaviour as the adolescent enters the post-15 years phase. One of the problems that clinicians face in making a diagnosis is that the *Diagnostic and Statistical Manual for Mental Disorders*, one of two psychiatric reference texts, uses criteria that are adult orientated rather than specific to adolescents or children. It is not that these criteria are incorrect but rather that they may be too narrow to cover adolescent behaviour (Pollack, 1999, p.320).

Once a decision has been made to intervene, medication and other talking treatments are indicated and often combined. Both counselling and cognitive behaviour therapy have proved to be effective when working with young people. Medication is often used although this needs to be carefully monitored as much less is known about the effect of this medication on children compared to adults. Indeed some medications, like some of the selective serotonin reuptake inhibitors (SSRIs) which are used extensively with adults, are not licensed for use on people under the age of 18 years as a result of considerable concern about possible side effects.

Hyperkinetic disorders or attention deficit hyperactivity disorder

Hyperkinetic disorder is the term used by British and European physicians when diagnosing attention deficit hyperactivity disorder/attention deficit disorder which it is claimed affects about 4% of the children and adolescents in the USA and a smaller but increasing percentage in the UK, estimated to be about 1%. In part this is as a result of psychiatrists in the UK adopting the more liberal diagnosis that is used in the USA. Signs include impaired functioning in situations where concentration is expected including classrooms and small group meetings. This can also manifest itself with impulsive behaviours and poor levels of functioning in relation to friends.

Interventions can either be medication, often Ritalin, or intensive behaviour modification or in some cases both. Ritalin is a psychostimulant and is from the same family as 'speed'. Although you would expect stimulants to make hyperactive young people more active it does in fact have the opposite effect for most young people.

Stimulant medication works for a short time and has the effect of helping the young person to concentrate and to work better at school as well as at home. Considerable gains in school performance and social ability have been reported. This medication works better when parent(s) are encouraged to provide practical and emotional support for their child. Stimulants are probably overused in the USA and underused in the UK and this medication is prescription only. Unfortunately in the US and increasingly in the UK it is reported that young people sell this medication to their classmates as it also acts as an appetite suppressant. Young people may also 'save up' their medication and take a lot at once to get the 'buzz'. Where stimulants have not worked doctors will often prescribe non-stimulant medication such as imipramine, fluoxetine or clonidine.

Social workers can provide behaviour management, counselling, and psychotherapy. Children and young people will inevitably experience low self-esteem and will be challenging to engage with in any meaningful way. Often parental attention is craved for, even when it is negative, and parents may need your help to learn how to reward positive behaviours and to ignore the negative behaviour. Children with hyperkinetic disorder benefit from being rewarded as much as anyone else even though their extreme behaviour can be especially difficult and demanding. This approach may be as effective as prescribing medication.

It is important that you work with not only the young person and their family but also the school so that everyone is aware of what the intervention is and their role in the treatment plan. Disruptive young people can develop expertise in manipulation and the art of playing off one party against the other.

Dissociative disorders

This condition affects a person's sense of who they are and the extent that they engage with reality. The result can be a feeling of being 'disconnected' from their social world. Everyone can feel this way from time to time; for example long-distance runners sometimes experience a 'high' as they float through a marathon, which could be considered similar. A similar experience can also occur as a result of the side effects of drugs or alcohol.

As you can imagine a diagnosis of dissociative disorder is controversial. However despite this it is likely that this disorder is much more common than previously thought. The diagnosis is often reached only after a series of several earlier misdiagnoses that can include borderline personality disorder and schizophrenia. The most complex of all of the dissociative disorders is known as dissociative identity disorder (DID) or multiple personality disorder in which the person experiences different personalities and often with an overlay of depression, severe mood swings, memory loss, anxiety and panic attacks.

The cause of this range of disorders is unclear but thought to include severe abuse in childhood and the lack of meaningful adult relationships that provide love and comfort. It is almost like the child or adolescent has had to be too self-reliant before they are capable of being so and has forgotten how to switch back to being a child. These disorders are diagnosed using some reliable tools such as the Dissociative Experiences Scale (DES) and the Structured Clinical Interview (SCID-D); a professional who is trained in this assessment tool must administer these. As with all mental disorders the cultural context needs to be uppermost in our minds when making such a diagnosis.

Social workers may work with people who have this disorder by providing information about self-help groups and by working with the person using a range of person-centred approaches. Self-help is often effective as are the various self-help groups and web sites that exist (listed at the end of this chapter).

Self-harm

Self-harm, or self-mutilation, has been estimated to affect as many as one in ten teenagers and is the intentional infliction of harm upon themselves. This can consist of excessive scratching, hitting, banging, biting, pinching or any other form of harming their body. However, most commonly it is cutting or burning themselves. It is important not to misinterpret these actions as suicidal gestures as they imply no intent of suicide (although in extreme cases these actions may result in accidental death).

There is a variety reasons as to why people would do this including self-punishment, to gain feelings of control, clearing their mind, expressing their psychological turmoil physically, seeking attention/manipulating others, and the adrenaline rush that the body naturally releases during these actions. Self-harm, when practised frequently, can escalate and become psychologically as well as physically addictive. The need to experience more severe harm in order to alleviate emotional pain and to attain an adrenaline rush is similar to the way that a heroin addict would use increasing amounts of heroin in order to feel the 'high' they initially felt. Due to this a reliance on self-harm may develop which is difficult to stop. It is important for them to form a new coping strategy to replace this addictive habit.

Eating disorders

Eating disorders involve serious disturbances of the 'normal' eating pattern, and an obsessive concentration on body size and diet. These disorders can be seen on a continuum from minimal intervention in the community through to life threatening conditions that require specialist residential services. Eating disorders are real, treatable mental disorders that can cause considerable distress to those who are experiencing the effects of the disorder and to their carers. (This is used as a case study later in this chapter.)

Social work interventions

Interventions range from working with families to individual work. You need to reflect on some of the value and ethical issues when working with young people. In Chapter 1 the issue of who is the primary client was raised which showed some potential conflicts of interest. In particular the dilemma of conformity with parental demands may be at the expense of the young person's emergent sense of self. Equally, working in an empowering way with the young person may be liberating for them but at the cost of their relationship with their parents and families.

Intervention can take many forms but family support is often the most common and most effective. This can consist of working with the family as a whole and/or working with individuals in the family. The thrust of government policy epitomised in the *Quality Protects* child and family consultation paper (DoH, 1999) is that early intervention by offering advice and support to parents will eventually reduce the number of people who at a young age are diagnosed as having a mental disorder (Walker, 1998).

The choice of intervention is considerable and it is important that services reflect service user needs rather than being resource driven. The following table sets out some of the main interventions that social workers and others might use, depending upon individual circumstances.

Type of intervention	Key aspects
Cognitive behaviour therapy (CBT)	Cognitive techniques challenging negative thoughts and behavioural techniques used to relieve maladaptive thoughts, beliefs and behaviours
Systemic and family therapy	Works on relationships within the family and patterns of interaction between the members
Interpersonal therapy (IPT)	Focuses on the interpersonal relationships of the service user; helps to improve communication patterns and how people relate to one another
Psycho-educational methods	This takes various forms and includes work with service users and families to help them to understand the nature of their disorder and how to promote their mental health
Counselling	Can take many different forms – usually one-to-one and gives the individual the opportunity to develop their understandings of their reactions to events

(Adapted from *Treatment Choice in Psychological Therapies and Counselling*. DoH, 2001)

There are occasions when a combination of interventions works; for example CBT and IPT are effective when working with people who are depressed and help to reduce the symptoms of depression (see above).

With the introduction of Every Child Matters: Change for Children the Government has set out a vision that will if fully enacted see a whole system transformation of children's service. This will be a comprehensive set of changes with the intention clearly set out on the five core ECM documents that set out the strategic planning and the ways in which services need to combine to safeguard vulnerable children. These documents are available on www.everychildmatters.gov.uk.

Of particular interest to you will be the guidance documents that support the effective delivery of services. These include establishing a common core of skills and knowledge, which covers the types of expertise that everyone, not just social workers, needs to possess when working with children, young people and families. It is clear that the government intends to ensure that the various agencies that have contact with children and young people need to work together in new ways to ensure children's services are more effective than at present.

This will include training all professionals who are working in primary care to develop assessment skills to help early identification of issues and emotional problems. The National Service Framework for Children in 2003 restated that children's mental health is everyone's business and set the aim of developing a comprehensive CAMHS service. This will see a rapid growth in training programmes that will try to increase the capacity of the workforce at all levels to be able to cope with these increased expectations.

One of the major features of this approach will be the Common Assessment Framework (CAF), which will be an assessment process that can be used by all the workers in children's services. This is a simplified pre-assessment checklist, a process for carrying out these assessments : a standardised form to record and to share with others. Details of this, including a standard assessment form can be easily found at www.everychildmatters.gov.uk/caf

Consider the following extract from this web site:

> *Training for integrated working will not just be about training staff on specific new processes, it will be one of the most important vehicles for bringing practitioners together, opening up discussions and facilitating change in practice within a local area. In addition, this training must be complementary, and able to be integrated into, the wider Every Child Matters: Change for Children programme and other initatives, especially training on the Common Core of Skills and Knowledge for the Children's Workforce.* (www.everychildmatters.gov.uk/caf)

Services for children and adolescents

Child and Adolescent Mental Health Services are organised into four tiers of service. These are important for professionals who are involved in this area of work to understand as is the connection between the various organisations who provide services for children and adolescents. This structure is set out below and is adapted from the *CAMHS Handbook* (DoH, 1995).

First tier: primary care

This is the level at which interventions are made by GPs, health visitors, school nurses teachers and social workers. The distinguishing feature of this tier is that it is generally provided by non-specialists who can work with children and adolescents in ways that are non-stigmatising but still open up the possibility of early recognition of mental distress. This level of service is usually provided at a local level wherever the professional works.

Second tier

This level of service is provided by a uni-professional group, which includes clinical child psychologists, educational psychologists, child psychiatrists, community child nurses and social workers. This tier offers specialist training for first tier workers and consultation for professionals and their families as well as outreach services where specialist services are not indicated and they also offer assessment for tiers three and four. This level of service is provided at a small number of locations within the community.

Third tier

At this level of service this is a specialist service for people who have more severe and complex disorders. This is typically a multi-disciplinary team often working in a community child mental health clinic or outpatient service. This will include social workers, child and adolescent psychiatrists, clinical psychologists, occupational therapists and art and music therapists.

Fourth tier

This offers access through assessment to child psychiatric services including day units and residential units including in-hospital services for children and adolescents who are in need of highly specialised services. These include services for people who are severely mentally ill or who are at risk of serious self-harm or suicide. These are the most specialised of services and likely to be provided at a supra-region level as not all districts can resource this level of expertise.

Compulsory admission to psychiatric hospital

The legal framework governing the admission to a hospital of children and young people is complex. The *Code of Practice* (MHA, 1983) devotes a chapter to the issues that apply to children and young people. The Mental Health Act does not put any age limit upon admission, recognition that in the extreme it may be necessary for such people to be admitted to hospital against their wishes. Most young people who go into hospital do so as a last resort and most will go in as an informal patient.

However, Part II of the Mental Health Act provides for compulsory detention where a young person has been assessed as having a legal form of mental disorder and who is seriously at risk. This is covered in Chapter 3 but in summary the sections of the Act that are used are:

- Section 2 for assessment and treatment for up to 28 days.

- Section 4 for an emergency where waiting for a second doctor would cause undue delay and permits detention until the second doctor arrives for up to 72 hours.

- Section 5 can allow for emergency detention when the young person is in hospital as an informal patient and threatens to leave and leaving is considered by a doctor (can hold for up to 72 hours) to put the young person or others at serious risk, or where a nurse considers it a risk and a doctor is not immediately available (can hold for up to six hours).

- Section 3 for inpatient treatment for up to six months in the first instance.

The Mental Health Act Commission produces regular reports about the monitoring of children and young people who are admitted to hospitals under compulsion. These show that during the period 1999–2001 over 1,000 children and young people were admitted to hospital under the Act and that over half of these admissions were to adult wards (Ninth Biennial Report, 2001). This is a particularly disappointing number as the government's CAMHS initiative was expected to reduce the number of people who need inpatient specialist services (Department of Health, 1998).

In this context it is important that all those concerned with the treatment of the young person should be able to let the young person and their family or carer know about the services that are available and their legal rights in respect of these.

If a child under the age of 16 is being admitted to hospital the following need to be considered:

- Who has parental responsibility? If the child has been subject to a court order it is important for those concerned with the treatment to have copies of these orders (residence order, care order, contact order, etc.).

- To determine the extent to which the child has the capacity to make his or her own decisions in terms of their emotional maturity, intellectual capacity and mental state.

- When a parent refuses treatment for their child to be able to evaluate the soundness of this decision.

- The range of alternatives to hospital admission and a risk assessment of them.

(Adapted from the *Code of Practice*, 1983, 31.4, a-e)

Children and adolescents who are socially excluded

This group has been identified for specific attention by the government which has set targets for excluding young people and provided funding for specific projects. Such children and young people could be from asylum seeker families, or refugees who may have been witness to considerable trauma, both of which can magnify their experiences of isolation and exclusion in the UK. Although commonsense tells us that such experiences must cause stress and that this can result in mental disorder there is no conclusive evidence. What we do know is that the stress of living in a family at the edges of society is in itself likely to cause mental health problems for members of the family including children. This will include the effects of physical and emotional abuse that may result from continual pressure and the isolation of parents. The impact of racism upon children and such families is under-researched but again it is likely that this is a compounding factor, which results in mental disorder for some young people.

Black and minority ethnic children are, like some of their adult counterparts, over represented in the mental health system. They may have suffered from developmental delay and other problems that are not of their making but may be a result of social exclusions and racism.

ACTIVITY 4.2

Imagine that you are have arranged for a young girl aged 14 to visit you at the office to discuss mental health problems that she has talked about with her teacher. Write down what factors you think are crucial to helping to build up a good relationship with her. e.g. provide a suitable setting.

The ideas that you might have come up with would include:

- *Having a suitable setting that is welcoming, private, safe, secure, has few distractions, materials to draw or write with, comfortable seating alongside each other.*

- *Plan the session and read the previous session's notes.*

- *Boundaries need to be set, identifying what will be discussed and what will not be discussed.*

- *Keeping an open mind is important to allow you to gather valid evidence with the young person acting as your guide.*

- *Listening and reflecting are basic interviewing skills for you to use to get as full a picture as possible about the young person's life and the analysis of their situation.*

- *Empathy and intuition, trying to walk in the young person's shoes, will help you to understand what is going on for the young person and how they assess their situation.*

- *Safety: always ensure that you are not left exposed to allegations about your conduct which may mean that you need to leave the room door open or interview with another colleague.*

(This list is adapted from Walker (2003) pp. 37–8)

Engaging and communicating with adolescents

Adolescents may be referred to you by their parent, teacher, or be seen by you as a result of other work that you are doing with the family. Adolescents are usually difficult to engage in any form of therapeutic work. Many professionals think that specialist mental health services only reach about 20% of adolescents who need these services. For all those adolescents who do reach out and engage there will be many more who will see you once or twice, and that will be enough and they disappear off your files. Of course it could be that even brief interventions can work and it can also be that a positive experience at least sets up the possibility of a return by the adolescent at some later stage.

However it may be important to help adolescents and young people early on in their lives to develop mechanisms that enable them to resolve difficulties that may adversely affect their mental health in later life. If adolescence is a time of transition between life stages it is also a time in which learning occurs about how to deal with the inevitable problems that life throws up. Faulty learning at this stage can result in longer-term mental health problems.

ACTIVITY **4.3**

From your experience write down what you think are some of the 'life events' that adolescents may have to deal with when growing up.

We can all draw upon our personal experiences and those of our friends when we went through this stage in our development. Ann Weal (1999) draws upon research to list some of these events which include:

- *conflict in the family;*
- *experience of being in care;*
- *poor development of verbal, literacy and academic skills;*
- *unmet emotional needs.*

To which you probably could have added bullying at school, peer pressure to look good, go to parties, have a boyfriend/girlfriend, have sex, not to have sex, etc. The list quickly grows and with it the potential for tension between competing demands.

Eating disorders

'Eating disorder' is a generic term that includes anorexia nervosa; bulimia and compulsive over-eating. These can develop into serious and often complex disorders that cause considerable anxiety and distress for the young person and their families. MIND estimate that one in 100 women in the UK between the ages of 15 and 30 experiences anorexia. Male representation is much smaller although growing in prevalence. (National Institute of Mental Health, 2001). Eating disorder is ranked as the third most chronic illness in female adolescents (USA brief notes on the mental health of children and adolescents, October 2003).

Anorexia nervosa affects teenagers, usually girls, who are typically perfectionists and have the potential to do well at school. They may have the additional diagnosis of obsessive compulsive disorder (OCD). They will typically have low self-esteem and may believe that they are fat even in the face of seemingly overwhelming evidence that they are emaciated. Many teens experience a fleeting sense of control when refusing food and may enjoy the food battleground that has been created with parents or carers.

Bulimia has different symptoms from anorexia and the teenager will typically binge on huge quantities of food and later eliminate the food through the use of powerful laxatives or self-induced vomiting. Such binges can be alternated with periods of diet. It can be hard for parents and others to discover bulimia as people become quite clever in concealing this condition as the adolescent may be of average weight (due to binging and then dieting). Also purging can occur with any food intake which although strictly would not be classified as bulimia is included as an eating disorder not otherwise specific (EDNOS) or atypical eating disorder.

In diagnostic terms adolescents are usually considered separately from adults as the strict diagnostic criteria of the DSM IV may not be entirely applicable to adolescents. For example adolescence is a time when there is wide variability in weight, height and sexual maturation as well as cognitive development which may make this diagnostic tool unreliable. This can result in some adolescents who have anorexia nervosa going undiagnosed (Society for Adolescent Medicine position paper, 2000.)

The treatment options depend upon the nature and development of the condition. Assessment needs to include clinical manifestations and social and psychological contexts. This is best carried out with an interdisciplinary team approach and may need to cover nutritional advice and counselling.

In a small number of instances there may need to be a period of hospitalisation followed by attendance at a day programme and a supported return to school or the community. The aim should be to provide a seamless transition from inpatient care to outpatient and to be person-centred.

What factors lie behind anorexia and other eating disorders?

A major study involving over 2,000 people in Australia has shown that those who previously dieted to a severe level were five times more likely to experience an eating disorder than those who dieted moderately. This led the research team to suggest that a safer way to control adolescent weight would be through an exercise programme and an educational input about diet and shape.

The connection between diet and the development of eating disorder is not made in every case. However:

> 'every morning hundreds and thousands of women wake up worrying about whether it is going to be a "good day" or a "bad day" in relation to food. They feel remorse for what they ate yesterday and hope that they will have more control today' (Orbach, 1986, p.1).

Orbach suggests that eating disorders, in particular anorexia nervosa, have become metaphors for the way in which society attempts to shape our lives and in this case the bodies of women. In this scenario women find themselves having to mediate their passions and desires, often in a public way, to achieve what they perceive as the desired physical shape. Thus eating can become a ready-made battleground on which women regularly seek to starve themselves to get closer to the perceived perfection of the catwalk model.

While anorexia, bulimia and compulsive overeating do not affect all women, the issues about shape and the centrality of food to the female experience mean that the issues about eating and the realities of eating disorder can be seen as an extreme manifestation of the inner turmoil that many women feel in relation to their bodies. Thus Orbach suggests that the adolescent girl must learn to develop a split between her body and the development of herself and that the girl fantasises over the benefits that might come her way with a slimmer body. This can be hard for men to appreciate and, especially, to understand the messages that men give out to women about their desirability.

There is no overall theory that can explain how this condition begins but there is agreement that stressful events can be seen as an intervening variable that might trigger off mental disorder (see Chapter 2 for a more detailed explanation). However eating disorders are not just about shape and diet, they can occur as the adolescent attempts to get control over their lives. The onset of the condition is sometimes linked to previous sexual abuse or other significant physical or psychological trauma. Another explanation is that it is the unconscious attempt by the young woman to stop her body developing during adolescence. All these ideas are interesting and of course relevant to our study and if you are going to work in this area or experience this condition yourself you will need to read more.

Although there is dispute over the actual cause of eating disorder there are some common factors. The most important of these is the way in which the person needs to feel in control of at least a part of their lives. People with eating disorders often feel that controlling their eating in such a severe manner is the only way that they can control their lives. Those on the outside, paradoxically, may see this as the ultimate expression of someone who has actually lost control of their lives.

This is primarily a condition that affects women, but the number of boys and men affected by eating disorders is on the increase. At present they account for about 10% of identified eating disorders (Neustatter, 2003). It is quite possible that as society becomes more obsessed with the human shape men are beginning to feel the pressure of being the ideal shape and that this striving for the unobtainable perfect body produces casualties on the way.

The social work response

Listening and trying to understand the person's experience and not jumping to conclusions that are not supported by evidence is key. People who experience this distress are often smart, self-critical and competitive people. They can be very able to discuss all aspects of their condition without getting down to the personal reasons about why they are that way and how they can begin to get a better balance in their lives. A review of the literature by Mark Griffith led him to conclude:

> *... and while it might not be possible to offer either an exhaustive nor evidence-based way forward, I think we can say that interventions in general, should be characterised by confidentiality, choice, and a determined effort to engage the adolescent's family.*
> (Griffiths,1998, p.10)

Lisa's story

This case study is based on the personal and professional experience of young people who I know and have worked with. I have altered the case to disguise their identities but without losing the essential features. It may surprise you to look at young people's narratives and to see just how many similarities there are between them.

For Lisa the arrival of anorexia was like the arrival of a person who lived inside her head and who had an alternative view of the world. This voice spoke deep down inside and said what to eat and what not to eat. At the age of 14 this voice came to live with Lisa. She couldn't remember the exact day but can recall that the effect was that this voice was struggling for control over her eating habits.

Lisa is a smart young woman who was self-critical and into alternative politics and protests.

At first Lisa was strong and felt that she was able to control the voice and argue with it when the instruction was to eat nothing. The struggle with the voice became very tiring. What do you say to those around you about the arrival of a voice? She was experiencing a degree of dissociation and in particular dissociative identity disorder with each identity assuming control at various times.

The easiest approach was to avoid eating with other people and to have a commitment to a harsh vegetarian diet. These combined made it more acceptable not to eat regular meals. She switched from school meals to a packed lunch, which she threw away. Gradually people around her, her family and friends, began to notice and it became a battleground at meal times. No one understood the struggle that was going on for her with her voice that she thought of as being evil but which no one else knew about. She wore several layers of loose-fitting clothes which hid her weight loss. These strategies concealed the loss of weight and the reality that she had become very skinny.

As Lisa began to lose weight and her skin and hair showed signs of poor nutrition she took the bold step of seeking help from the school and a referral was made to the educational psychologist. At this point she was in a poor frame of mind, worn out by the battles with the voice and lacking in energy. One night she took a large quantity of anti-depressants, paracetamol and anything else that was to hand all washed down with a large quantity of vodka.

Discovered by her mother she was admitted to the accident and emergency unit and given life-saving treatment. The following day she was transferred to a specialist unit. Here she was able to have her eating carefully monitored and to receive specialist input from the team, which included a child and adolescent psychiatrist, psychologist and social worker. She went to a 'group' where she learnt that others had experienced similar situations and also had voices that sought to control their food intake and kept telling them that they were overweight.

The support of the other young people in the unit was especially helpful and contrasted with the general lack of understanding in the world outside of the unit. The unit brought together her immediate family once a week for a Saturday group where attempts were made to help the family recognise the difficulties that Lisa faced and the family's role in this. It was here that the family learnt not to keep on at Lisa for not eating and that trying to persuade her to put on weight was making the situation worse rather than better. It was difficult for the family to accept that Lisa was not doing this to hurt the family but was engaged in a struggle that was hers alone and that the most helpful approach was for them to listen to Lisa, try to understand and to offer their support.

Over a period of a few weeks Lisa got into a position where she pushed the voice into the background and learned some techniques that helped her to keep it there. She was also prescribed anti-depressants and a mood stabiliser from her psychiatrist. Every morning she was weighed and her weight gains recorded. Any loss meant reduction in privileges and closer attention being paid to her diet, a process that she resented but deep down knew helped.

Today Lisa continues to have mental health problems but the eating component of her disorder is at least under control and the eating voice has subsided. Now that she has a more understanding family she can draw some strength from this support although she realises that outside of a small circle there are few people who will understand what she has been through.

Early Intervention

Early warning signs are important to recognise and early intervention may well have prevented Lisa's later hospitalisation. Tiers one and two are usually the first point of service and late referrals can be put down to families and friends mistaking signs of mental health stress as 'natural' or 'normal behaviour' for adolescents. Among the general signs are the following:

Emotional signs
- Sad or anxious without apparent reason and for unusually long periods of time;
- constant concern about appearance;
- feelings of worthlessness.

Behavioural signs
Look for behaviour that has changed recently or causes comment by others:
- poor concentration;
- nightmares/insomnia;
- loss in women of menstrual cycle;
- sudden and unexplained significant weight loss;
- alcohol or drug misuse including laxatives;
- self-induced vomiting;

- concern about diet and calorie counting;

- wants to be alone;

- over-exercising;

- light-headedness and/or fainting;

- evidence of purging.

Recognising early signs

All the above need to be put into the context that change is a 'normal' part of adolescence. Equally, families may be reluctant to seek help fearing the negative effects of labelling of their child. Ignoring early signs of mental health problems in children and young people can have detrimental long-term effects. Early intervention will mean working at the preventative level with young people before their mental health problems become mental disorder.

In Lisa's case several factors were noted as set out below:

- Her parents had divorced and there was still considerable acrimony between them. Lisa was often caught up in the middle of these battles and having to make judgments about competing demands.

- Several friends had noticed that she was more and more withdrawn and spent less time in company and more time on her own listening with headphones to her music.

- She was becoming more obsessive about a number of things including dietary needs, likes and dislikes.

- Her schoolwork had fallen well below her previous level and certainly below what the teachers thought that she was capable of achieving (in some cases there is a sudden dramatic increase in grades).

Tier one services could have helped at this stage and avoided the risk of stigma and labelling that a late referral to the specialist might bring. Increasingly social workers are being located in schools and colleges, which can help mobilise an early response. The Connexions service has Personal Advisors often located in schools who can also provide easy access to services at levels one and two.

ACTIVITY **4.4**

You are a social worker placed in a secondary school. Lisa's friends have come to see you as they are concerned about her. What action would you take? Think about this using the 'assessment framework'. Would you:

- *talk to Lisa;*

- *talk to Lisa's parents;*

- *talk to Lisa's teachers and others at the school?*

Depending upon what happened with your preliminary assessment it might be appropriate to refer Lisa for supportive counselling and/or put her in touch with a self-help group. There are also numerous websites that are great sources of information and which Lisa might want to visit. You should check out what your local CAMHS website is.

Interventions

There are two types of interventions, those that are called **psychological therapies** and those that are **clinical interventions** and these are summarised below. Like work with adults the emphasis needs to be on provision of a multi-disciplinary approach that is evidence based. Before using any form of intervention you should check the evidence to see what works best in what situation and what skill level is needed to engage with service users.

Psychotherapy

Psychotherapy focuses upon our inner world and through a process of insight development, usually on a one to one basis, helps to develop a greater awareness of the nature of an eating disorder and to understand possible causes. Through this understanding people are in a better position to get control over their eating disorder. The theoretical position of this intervention is based in the work of Freud, Klein and Piaget. This form of intervention is usually undertaken by psychologists, psychiatrists or a counsellor and can cover all tiers of CAMHS although usually this intervention is at tiers one and two.

Cognitive behaviour therapy

This focuses not on the inner world of the young person but on the actual behaviours. Here the cause is less important than the manifestation of the behaviours and there is a belief that the causes may not be able to be changed but the behaviours can be altered. The therapist or social worker will work with the person to help them to identify negative and counter-productive thoughts and replace them with a more positive frame of mind. Usually used at tiers one and two.

Psycho-social intervention

This draws upon theoretical positions that are founded in the social sciences and see the person in a social context allowing for intervention that recognises the importance of empowering interventions. Here social workers play a crucial part as they are unique in being able to work with the service user. By so doing they can understand what is happening to the service user and to recognise and intervene to provide access to self-help groups, advocacy, etc. Usually a tiers one and two intervention.

Alternative therapies

These are widely available, often in local community centres or in specialist agencies like MIND, but are increasingly also available for inpatient treatment. These therapies help the person to find alternative ways of expressing themselves through movement, dance, art, poetry and music. There are also a number of self-help texts that some service users report as being very helpful (see further reading). Usually a tier one service but can be across all tiers.

Inpatient

In an extreme case of eating disorder the person's health can be at serious risk as weight loss and nutritional imbalances reach life-threatening proportions. This is tiers three and four and requires a whole-team approach if the condition is to be reversed before long-lasting damage occurs. Specialist clinics are available which may operate under specific therapeutic regimes. Any programme of treatment should form part of a person's agreed care programme (*Code of Practice*, 18, p. 87) and all treatments should follow a full discussion of the form that the treatment will take, and how and when it will be reviewed.

In some cases young people may be 'force fed' under the Mental Health Act (1983) and social workers may be required to sign the legal forms as a person not connected directly with the treatment of the patient but one who knows that patient's circumstances.

Stress busting tips

Managing stressful distractions when trying to study

One of the main problems when trying to get down to serious study is the inner dialogue, which goes on in our minds and keeps playing messages like 'I cannot do this' or 'I am not clever enough' or 'I'd rather do — well anything but this.' Avoidance of hard work like learning seems to be part of a common human condition but using some principles from cognitive therapy can help you to alter these inner conversations and by so doing reduce the impact of stress.

How to turn down the inner voice volume

- Close your eyes.

- Listen to all those negative words until they become clear.

- Imagine this is like a radio – reach out and turn the volume up.

- Listen and make sure that the voices in your head do become louder.

- ENJOY YOUR CONTROL.

- Reach out and turn down the volume – notice how the voices go lower.

- Continue until the sounds become distant and resemble the gentle murmur of the ocean on a still day.

- The sound is still there only now you cannot even make out the words.

- Practise this technique so that managing these internal conversations becomes easier each time that you use this technique.

This method of stress busting requires practice and can be effective for you. With care and skill it can also be used when working with adolescents who are struggling to engage with school.

Steven Walker, (2003) *Social Work and Child and Adolescent Mental Health.* Lyme Regis: Russell House.

This is one of the few and certainly the best reads in this area. In this book you will find many of the ideas in this chapter covered in more depth. All chapters are good but Chapter 7 on socially inclusive practice is relevant to this area of work and pulls together the recent government ideas and gives out ideas for a broad ranging practice that works to combat the worst effects of social exclusion.

Grainne Smith *Anorexia and Bulimia in the Family: One Parent's Practical Guide to Recovery* (2004). Chichester: Wiley:

This is a practical guide, written by a parent whose daughter experienced anorexia, and is good reading as it combines practical advice with latest research.

Useful organisations

MIND – The mental health charity that provides a voice for people with mental health distress and disorder. It also has a range of fact sheets and publications that make essential reading for those who want more information about mental health. It also runs a number of supportive workshops and user groups. This could be your first port of call for alternative health care, information and/or support. www.mind.org.uk

Dissociative disorder

Useful websites include:
www.dissociation.co.uk
A resource for professionals.

www.mosaicminds.org
A website that offers assistance for survivors of childhood trauma and has a particular focus on dissociative disorder.

www.ukssd.org
This is the UK society for the study of dissociation.

Eating disorders

Eating Disorders Association offers help and support for people who experience eating disorder.
Young person's helpline: 01603 765050.
www.edauk.com

Overeaters Anonymous. Although based in Manchester this organisation runs local groups for compulsive overeaters. Tel: 07000 784985.

Pale Reflections is a popular website for adolescents who find the material accurate and informative. This is a USA site.
www.pale-reflections.com

Association for Dance Movement Therapy. Promotes dance therapy and can provide lists of locally based qualified therapists.
Email enquiries to dance.voice@cableinet.co.uk

The Institute for Optimum Nutrition. Sells books, tapes and videos and can refer callers to nutritionists throughout the country. Tel: 020 8877 9993
Email allion@ion.ac.uk

The Mental Health Act Commission publishes a series of Guidance Notes among which is the technical and detailed Note No. 3 on *Guidance and Treatment of Anorexia Nervosa under the Mental Health Act 1983* which was published in August 1997. Tel: 0115 943 7100

ADD/ADHD Family Support Group UK offers support for families. Tel: 01373 826045

A great website is provided by the Royal College of Psychiatrists – www.rcpsych.ac.uk – which has information sheets that cover many of the topics in this chapter.

YoungMinds, 102–8 Clerkenwell Road, London EC1M 5SA. Tel: 020 7336 8445
www.youngminds.org.uk

National Institute of Mental Health
www.nimh.nih.gov/publicat/eatingdisorder.cfm

National Institute of Mental Health (2001) *Eating disorder: facts about eating disorders and the search for solutions*. A detailed booklet describing symptoms, causes, and treatment, with information on getting help and coping.

Chapter 5

Working with vulnerable people: adults who are short-term service users

A C H I E V I N G   A   S O C I A L   W O R K   D E G R E E

This chapter will help you to meet the following National Occupational Standards.

Key Role 1: Prepare for and work with individuals, families, carers, groups and communities to assess their needs and circumstances

- Assess needs and options to recommend a course of action.

Key Role 2: Plan, carry out, review and evaluate social work practice, with individuals, families, carers, groups and communities and other professionals

- Interact with individuals, families, carers, groups and communities to achieve change and development and to improve life opportunities.
- Address behaviour which presents a risk to individuals, families, carers, groups and communities.

Key Role 6: Demonstrate professional competence in social work practice

- Research, analyse, evaluate and use current knowledge of best social work practice.
- Work within agreed standards of social work practice and ensure own professional development.

It will also introduce you to the following academic standards as set out in the subject benchmark statement which includes:

2 Defining principles

2.2.1 Social work is located within different social welfare contexts.

2.2.2 There are competing views in society at large on the nature of social work and on its place and purpose.

2.4 Social work is a moral activity that requires practitioners to make and implement difficult decisions about human situations that involve the potential for benefit or harm.

3 Knowledge, understanding and skills

3.1.1 Social work services and service users

The nature and validity of different definitions of, and explanations for, the characteristics and circumstances of service users and the services required by them.

The relationship between agency policies, legal requirements and professional boundaries in shaping the nature of services provided in inter-disciplinary contexts and the issues associated with working across professional boundaries and within different disciplinary groups.

3.1.2 The service delivery context

The issues and trends in modern public and social policy and their relationship to contemporary practice and service delivery in social work.

The significance of interrelationships with other social services, especially education, housing, health, income maintenance and criminal justice.

The current range and appropriateness of statutory, voluntary and private agencies providing community-based, day-care, residential and other services and the organisational systems inherent within these.

> **3.1.3 Values and ethics**
> The moral concepts of rights, responsibility, freedom, authority and power inherent in the practice of social workers as moral and statutory agents.
> **3.1.4 Social work theory**
> Research-based concepts and critical explanations for social work theory.
> The characteristics of practice in a range of community-based and organisational settings including group care, within statutory, voluntary and private sectors.

The liberty of the individual must be thus far limited; he must not make himself a nuisance to other people.
John Stuart Mill (1859)

Introduction

This chapter introduces some of the key concepts and skills that are needed for the social work role in times of short-term acute need. It builds on the learning that has occurred in earlier chapters. The role of the primary care teams is covered and the need for liaison with other professionals in this area is reinforced. Although there are different approaches when working with service users who have chronic as opposed to acute conditions there are also overlaps between the two and today's short-term user could develop into tomorrow's long-term user. To help you to unravel all of this an illustrative example is used throughout based on an older person who experiences depression.

Assessment of people who pose a risk to themselves is a complex and difficult task whether they live in the community or are hospitalised. If they live in the community one of the goals will be to achieve a balance between providing good quality intervention and avoidance of unnecessary risks. Admission to hospital is used as an example to help you to understand when this is necessary.

A case example is used to show how social workers may need to work with a service user who is potentially suicidal. This highlights key areas such as community care and direct payments.

Emphasis is placed in this chapter on assessment for services and the imaginative use of resources. This will cover how social workers can work with providers to provide 24-hour crisis support services.

Policy context

The statistics

Suicide is one of the major causes of death in England, Wales and Scotland and accounts for approximately 15% of all deaths annually although the exact numbers are unclear due in part to the reluctance sometimes of coroners to find a verdict of suicide. This is partly due to the varying criteria but also because of respect for the families. Thus it is quite likely that this figure of 15% is an under-representation of the actual number of suicides. This means that every year about 4,000 people in England, Wales and Scotland kill themselves. In this figure you will find that men outnumber women by about 2:1 and the main concern is for young men in the 15–24 age range and elderly people over the age of 74 (Williams and Morgan, 1994).

National targets

Suicide reduction
The national suicide prevention strategy for England Our Healthier Nation (OHN) was launched in 2002 with the clear if ambitious aim of reducing the death rate from suicide by at least a fifth by the year 2010. Suicide rates overall have shown a downward trend since the 1980s and in 1995/6/7 they were estimated to be 9.2 deaths for each 100,000 population and the 2005 figures show that this is now down to 8.6 deaths per 100,000 well on route to acheiving the 7.3 deaths per 100,000 target in 2009/10/11 (NIMHE, 2006).

The Department of Health monitors these targets and the good news is that they are falling slowly and it is likely that targets will be met. It is also important to learn about the circumstances in which people kill themselves and this is also the subject of official investigation.

The Confidential Inquiry
The Department of Health has established a Confidential Inquiry into Homicides and Suicides by Mentally Ill People, to try to identify more precisely the causes of death and the circumstances surrounding death. This Inquiry has been led by the Royal College of Psychiatry and reports will be published from time to time. The first report was in 1996 and described the detailed examination of 240 suicides of which 154 were outpatients. There are numerous findings but among these are that the most common life event before suicide was the breakdown of a marriage or partnership, followed by: bereavement; physical illness and financial problems (adapted from Eldergill, 1998). Relevant to our case example is the finding that over half the people who had committed suicide had contact with the services the week prior to that event.

Workforce
The National Institute for Mental Health England (NIMHE) National Workforce programme has set some priorities for the modern mental health service that includes developing national capacity for work with service users in the community.

By mid 2006 there are the following:

- 343 crisis resolution teams to provide intensive support;

- 262 assertive outreach teams to provide intensive support for difficult to engage service users;

- 109 early intervention teams to carry out assessment and care for service users who are experiencing the first onset of psychosis (adapted from NIMHE Annual Report, 2006).

Workforce developments:

- 500 community mental health 'gateway' workers;

- 700 additional staff to support carers.

By the end of 2006 the aim was that the workforce capacity would be further developed and the shift from doctors to other healthcare professionals, including social workers and the greater involvement of support staff (NIMHE, 2003).

Now we should make the move from policy to application and consider the case of Mr Skeffling (this is his preferred mode of address). This case is used throughout the remainder of this chapter to show how assessment and intervention can be made and what research and statute should inform the kind of decisions that you as the social worker would be making with the service user.

CASE STUDY

Phase one
Mr Skeffling lives with his wife in a remote country village. He is 68 years old and she is 69 and they have lived in the same area for the last 20 years or so. They have two children, both adults, who live in cities some 55 miles away. Mr Skeffling has become depressed and has been prescribed anti-depressants by his GP. Mrs Skeffling returned home after visiting her son for a couple of days to find her husband in a very distressed state. At first she was unsure if he had been drinking heavily but he eventually told her that he had taken a large amount of his medication all at once and washed it down with his favourite whisky. He said that he was 'absolutely fed up with life – it was all too much and he had had enough'. She called her doctor who made arrangements for Mr Skeffling to be admitted informally to the local psychiatric unit.

The admission to hospital was made in order to provide Mr Skeffling with an environment that could respond to the immediate risk and assess the next step. A referral is made to the community mental health team and as the social worker you visit first thing the following morning. By this time Mr Skeffling has settled and is feeling somewhat embarrassed by in his view 'all the fuss about nothing'. He knows that in the last few months he has been very down, isn't very happy with the diagnosis of depression but wants to go back home as soon as possible.

Depression and suicide

How common is mental disorder among older people? Depression in old age is far more common than many people think. Various estimates suggest that as many as 10% of people aged over 65 experience depression that is sufficient to warrant the involvement of professionals (Mental Health Foundation, 2004). More women are affected than men. Other severe forms of mental disorder are also prevalent including of course the organic form known as dementia. When you consider that in England we are experiencing an ageing population the actual number of older people with mental disorder is gradually rising. There are about ten million people of pensionable age in the UK which is over 20% of the population at large. The number of people over 85 has shown a dramatic increase to the point where in 2001 they were 2% of the population or over one million people.

If you work through these figures you will realise that we are talking big numbers and estimates of one million older people experiencing depression are not far short of reality. But can depression be linked to suicide? The obvious answer is yes, but this does need some careful examination before assuming that one necessarily leads to another. First the reality is that the highest suicide rate is found among elderly people and in particular those over 75. This is still the case even though the actual total number of people who successfully kill themselves has begun to fall in recent years.

General practitioners are at the front line when it comes to recognising depression in people. In the case of older people, depression can be overlooked if the GP wrongly thinks that older people are unlikely to be depressed and instead perhaps concentrates on physical problems. Identifying ways of differentiating depression from the effects of older age, which could include sleep disturbance; lowering of activity levels; lower libido and/or greater level of fatigue presents a challenge for practitioners. There are a number of specialist rating scales that help the professional recognise the symptoms of depression and make this task easier and more valid. These include the Geriatric Depression Scale (GDS) (Ulas and Connor, 1999). Like most disorders early recognition usually offers the best chance for good recovery.

Traditionally services are organised in tiers or levels with access to the higher tiers being through the referral system. Primary care is the first tier with services being provided by the GP and other professionals. The general principle is that people's mental health needs should be met at the lowest tier possible and this will involve other agencies such as social services and the voluntary sector.

Social factors

> ### CASE STUDY *continued*
>
> *After a week in hospital Mr Skeffling returns home agreeing to take the anti-depressant medication and to work with the team to develop the care plan into a more comprehensive one. As the social worker you will take on the role of care coordinator/key worker. This includes visiting him at his home.*
>
> *After two interviews with the couple it is becoming clear that their relationship is not especially strong and that Mr Skeffling feels ignored and isolated. Whereas at one time he was a full-time farm worker he is now retired and on a fixed and modest retirement income. His best friend died last year which has left him with a sense of despair.*

What factors contribute to depression? The psycho-social model, suggested in Chapter 2, helps to identify possible factors and for Mr Skeffling in particular the importance of loss to him. His close friend and really only male friend in the last 20 years has been his near neighbour who died seven months ago. The two of them shared an interest in going to the nearby village pub in the neighbour's car and enjoyed the atmosphere and watching live football matches. Mr Skeffling has been once or twice since but felt very isolated and thought that everyone was looking at him. The only time that he gets out is to go shopping in the nearby town which he finds uninteresting.

Although Mr and Mrs Skeffling have been married for a long time they appear to have got bored with each other's company and when together they frequently niggle at each other. He is critical of how his wife spends her time and their money while she complains that he is taking root in front of the television. Whereas his wife has a circle of female friends whom she meets twice a week in the church hall Mr Skeffling doesn't have anyone to talk to or to confide in.

As a further complicating factor Mr Skeffling's car is playing up and will need major repairs or replacing soon. They both say that they cannot afford a new car or to spend a lot on the repair of their present one. Yet without the car they will be unable to go shopping or to make the odd trip to the town. Their children are adults who live quite a distance from them and only get to visit once a month at best and without a car the couple will not be able to go and see them.

CASE STUDY *continued*

The assessment of the situation that the couple find themselves in is starting to take shape. You should now see what factors you have identified as important from the above illustrative example and the notes afterwards.

The importance of loss as a significant factor in the onset of depression will probably be the first that you picked up. In this case it is a double hit as not only did Mr Skeffling lose his activity but also the only person with whom he appeared to have a close, confiding relationship.

Social work and suicide

Not all suicides are associated with mental disorder although the presence of a severe mental disorder increases the risk of suicide. It has been estimated that of the people who do commit suicide 90% experience mental disorder of some type and of these about 30% have expressed clear intent to kill themselves and 25% are psychiatric outpatients. This presents a real challenge to mental health teams. We now need to examine what factors need to be considered in Mr Skeffling's case.

Colin Pritchard describes various ways of estimating suicide risk and uses the Lettieri scale for older men which pinpoints the following key factors:

1. Recent serious loss.

2. Depression.

3. Element of anger or aggression in their behaviour.

4. Refusal to accept help.

5. Previous suicidal or self-harming history.

6. Failure in a major role of their lives.

(Adapted from Pritchard, 1995)

These represent what might be termed 'negative factors' and if you relate this to Mr Skeffling you can see that numbers 1, 2, 4 and 6 are present in varying degrees. This Lettieri scale is one of a number of measuring tools that assist in the prediction of suicide among the population. There are also several self-assessment scales that are in use. They vary in their clinical usefulness and the main use is to aid decision-making but not to replace it.

It is necessary to distinguish between risk of suicide in the short term and risk in the longer term. It has been estimated that about 2% of those who had one attempt will succeed within a year of the first attempt with a particular risk occurring in the first three months (see Butler and Pritchard, 1983). The difficulty that social workers and other clinicians have is assessing just who are the people who fall into this category. This requires a balance between identifying those most likely to be at risk while not intervening unnecessarily with those who are considered to be a lesser risk.

An additional approach is to work with the service user to help identify with them the positive factors or the 'reasons for living'. This approach assumes that the service user will be able, with help, to identify reasons for their life and to be able to put these alongside the more negative attributes. This helps you to work with the service user to identify their strengths or assets rather than only weaknesses or deficits.

ACTIVITY 5.1

Write down what you would consider to be the reasons for living that would be relevant for you and then write down what you think Mr Skeffling might say and compare the two.

I hope that you found plenty to put down for yourself. I think that Mr Skeffling would struggle a little with this and probably need prompting but he might list:

- hope that life will change;

- love of his family;

- being scared of the act of suicide;

- moral objections about suicide;

- a view that suicide is a sign of weakness.

(Adapted from Linehan, 1985 in Pritchard, 1995)

Working with people who have attempted suicide

The most important contribution that you can make as a social worker is to manage to work alongside your health colleagues to provide a joint approach yet retaining the essential and unique features of social work. A major concern when working with people who have attempted suicide is how or perhaps even if this should be discussed. There are many excellent texts about working with people who are at risk of suicide or serious self-harm.

In our case the psychiatrist at the unit will have carried out an assessment and this will have been discussed at the care planning meeting that will have taken place before discharge took place. The type of questions would include the following:

Questions about the incident itself:

- What was his intent?

- What is the relationship between his depression and this attempt?

- What is the risk at the present of a further attempt?

- What kind of help would he be willing to accept?

CASE STUDY *continued*

Mr Skeffling denies that this was a serious attempt. He has been suffering from mild to moderately severe depression for the last few months but also admitted that he has not been taking his medication regularly. No particular event led to the attempt but he describes it as a build up of events such as the death of his friend and the increased isolation that he feels. He is willing to work with the team to seek ways of improving his life. This would put him in the low risk category.

Questions about the degree of intent

- Was the attempt planned or impulsive?

- Did he know that he would be found soon after the attempt?

- What drugs were taken? How much alcohol was taken? Were there other drugs that were around but not taken?

- Was a suicide note left?

CASE STUDY *continued*

Mr Skeffling's attempt at suicide was not thought through and it appears impulsive. He used his prescription medication as the means of trying to 'end it all' and chose a time when his wife was out but also not long before he knew that she was going to return. No arrangements for following his death, suicide notes, or update of his will, were evident. These put the likelihood of suicide in the low to moderate category.

Assessment of current problems

- Relationship with family members;

- Financial status;

- Social networks, support isolation;

- General health;

- Use of alcohol or drugs.

The above is adapted from a number of guides to assessment (Butler and Pritchard, 1983; Eldergill, 1998; Pritchard, 1995).

CASE STUDY *continued*

Mr Skeffling's relationship with his wife has worsened over the last few years and he has no other person in whom to confide. He is struggling to get by financially and in particular is really anxious about living where they do and being without a car. His wife has a strong network of friends but most of his have either died or left the area. He does drink at home by himself from time to time and when he does it is often to excess. He is not very optimistic about the future. This puts him in the moderate risk category.

The use of such assessment tools should only be undertaken by someone who is skilled and experienced in their application. They are in common use and different clinicians favour different tools. Eldergill has drawn together some of the research findings in this field and some of these are set out below.

Source	Research findings
J.H.J. Bancroft and P. Marsack, *British Journal of Psychiatry* (1977) 131,394	The risk of completed suicide is increased where there is the presence of mental disorder and alcoholism
A.R. Beisser and J.E. Blanchette, *Diseases of the Nervous System* (1961) XXII, 7, 365–9	The risk of another suicide attempt is most common within three months of the first attempt
S. Ganzler, et al., *Life-Threatening Behaviour* (1971) 1, 184–202	A significant link can be made between attempted suicide attempts and social deprivation
N. Kreitman, *Parasuicide* (John Wiley, 1980)	1–2% of people who attempt suicide kill themselves within 12 months

(Adapted from Eldergill, 1998, p.733)

These research findings need to be put alongside other findings such as:

Safer Services, (1991). National Confidential Inquiry into Suicide and Homicide	Half the people who committed suicide had contact with mental health services in the week prior to the event
	At the last contact 85% were assessed as being low risk
Obafunwa and Busuttil, 1994	30% of all suicides are carried out by people who have seen their family doctor less than three weeks before they took their lives
Modestein and Schwarzenbach, 1992	Non-compliance in taking the prescribed medication is an indicator of risk

All research should be treated in a critical manner but also needs to be carefully considered and referred to by professionals. This is how professionals continually develop yet there is evidence that suggests that while medical practitioners may consult the research as a matter of course this is not the case with other professionals such as social workers.

Risk assessment

The evaluation of the above risk factors needs to be undertaken by a clinician who will weigh these up against the research. In the case of Mr Skeffling his behaviour appears to be more of a response to the present situation and discontent with his social isolation and financial situation than total despair with his life. Mrs Skeffling is on paper a viable carer but their relationship is difficult and more likely to be part of the problem rather than the solution. He has only recently seen the doctor for depression and at the time this was assessed as being mild. Since the initial emergency call out Mr Skeffling appears to be less despairing and to have appreciated the opportunity to talk though his worries with someone who is outside of the family.

ACTIVITY **5.2**

Look back at the developing case of Mr Skeffling and jot down what you think are the risk factors. What role could Mrs Skeffling play in the situation?

Policy background

The late 1980s and the 1990s witnessed the move from a policy that was focused upon long-stay hospital care to one that focused upon the provision of services in the community. The closure of large psychiatric hospitals and their community replacements meant that health and social services in many instances had to learn to work together and this is still an ongoing process. This theme ran throughout many government policy documents with suitably aspirational titles like *Building Bridges* (DoH, 1998); *Partnerships in Action* (DoH, 1998); Modernising Social Services (1998); and *Modernising Mental Health Services* (see DoH, 2002).

Care in the community – expanding services to offer choice

The mental health service as it is evolving has the idea of choice as a central and defining feature. By offering service users choice they can be better matched to appropriate services depending upon their need. That present day services are unresponsive, in many instances, to service user need is generally accepted but in order to have choice there would need to be an excess of supply over demand which seriously impacts on service efficiency. Thus services continually come up against the stark financial realities and it has proved difficult for services that are genuinely user-focused to be developed. To offer genuine choice means starting not with what services can be matched but what the service user needs. This requires innovation on the part of service providers and the imagination of those charged with assessment and planning (Onyett, 1992). It also means considerable resources need to be poured into making community care a positive choice that will enhance the lives of vulnerable people.

The key statute relating to care in the community is the National Health Service and Community Care Act 1990 which actually came into being in 1993. This Act has since been supplemented by The Carers (Recognition and Services Act) 1995, which introduced the right for carers to have an assessment of their needs made alongside the service user's assessment. The Community Care (Direct Payments) Act 1996 also enabled local authorities to provide cash for service users to enable them to purchase the kind of services that they want. The later HSCA 2001 made it a duty from April 2003 for local authorities not just to offer direct payments but extended the coverage to include people of any age. However even with all this legislation community care remains patchy and in many instances problematic.

CASE STUDY *continued*

Mr Skeffling has returned home and an assessment has been carried out to determine if he is eligible for community care services. It is quite clear that his wife, who is unable to drive, is unable and unwilling to take responsibility for her husband's well-being. She is very frightened that he might do something silly to himself.

Getting help depends first on having a Community Care Assessment that meets the 'eligibility criteria'. The assessment places service users into one of the following bands: critical, substantial, moderate or low. The assessment is a full one and may take time to organise and carry out but this does not prevent services from being provided or payments made until this occurs. Too often the assessment is about eligibility for existing services and how best they can be packaged to suit the service user instead of working with the service user to identify what would work well for them and a genuine assessment of need. Any assessment ought to look not only at what is missing but also the strengths of the service user and their individual environment.

The criteria that are used may vary slightly from area to area but will include some of the following in order to be put into the critical band:

- significant health problems have developed or will develop;
- inability to carry out vital personal care or domestic routines;
- social support systems and relationships cannot or will not be sustained;
- family and other social roles and responsibilities cannot or will not be undertaken;
- engagement with vital formal support systems is not being maintained;
- serious risk of harm to self or others exists;
- inability to access community facilities.

CASE STUDY *continued*

From what you have read about Mr Skeffling use the above list to check out if he meets any of the criteria and the level of importance to him.

The extent that he meets the above is largely dependent upon how you see the situation. This is an important point for assessments need to conform with equal opportunities which means taking time and approaching the assessment with the service user and others (if appropriate). Work like this needs skill, patience and transparency and the assessment should be signed off by all interested parties.

In the above activity it is likely that he meets all of those criteria but the question is the extent to which these are seen as vital or significant. Allocating assessment to bands is the next step to decide if he is eligible for community care services. In our example Mr Skeffling may just about meet the social services eligibility criteria at least in the short term.

What services can be provided?

Services will be provided to people who are unable to perform one or more basic tasks of daily living where:

a. informal support (Mrs Skeffling) cannot be reasonably expected to provide them;

b. service users (or their carers) are at significant risk without the provision of such services; or

c. services are clearly aimed at increasing independence.

Services will be provided to:

a. meet essential personal, social and educational needs;

b. ensure that service users and/or carers are not left at significant risk;

c. support carers to continue in their caring role;

d. support people to continue living in the community through a programme of rehabilitation.

Most councils have set up a direct payment support service of some sort to help people purchase their own services and to assist them with the legal obligations of employing personal assistants and accounting for the money. The scheme was widely extended in April 2003, which has resulted in a large increase in take up. Local authorities now have a duty to offer direct payments.

Support and self-help

The scheme that came into being is Direct Payments (Community Care (Direct Payments) Act 1996) that allows service users who are disabled, including people who have mental disorder, to receive cash payments in place of services from social services. The intention is that they will support service users who wish to remain independent but the use has been very restricted (Robbins, 2004). This approach was built on the views of what service users want and it was apparent that they wanted:

> ... *Information, help with ordinary living, support with personal growth and development. They want well co-ordinated packages of treatment, and a plan that takes account of their aspirations for the future.*
> (Robbins, pp.2–3)

The Direct Payments scheme offers another alternative that could be very empowering for the service user. When it was originally launched it had age restrictions and close relatives could not be paid. Unsurprisingly take up was low and these restrictions were removed with the HSCA (2001) legislation. The recipient is also responsible for managing and accounting for the money, which in turn most likely will require assistance and/or training.

ACTIVITY 5.3

Check out on the internet what information your local social care provider gives to potential mental health users. Putting in the key words 'direct payments' into a search engine such as Google will give you lots of information. If you had a mental disorder would you know where to go to get information and once you have the information would you want to have these payments? Although you might be eligible the thought of having to administer money yourself and to keep accurate and verifiable records may in themselves be a deterrent and turn you away from the direct payment solution. Most local authorities have websites for direct payments although these can be out of date.

Alternatives to traditional hospital based services

Acute and crisis services are designed to respond to a crisis and offer treatment that is less restrictive and less stigmatising than hospitalisation. The development of a range of options, although slow, is happening where government has taken the lead. The present day emphasis on a mixed economy of providers does not in itself produce variety. As smaller community based units proliferate the danger is that what is created is simply smaller hospitals, which are of course less efficient than a larger hospital that is provided by a single provider. The government has increased the level of funding that is available to mental health services to help finance diverse provision.

ACTIVITY 5.4

If you had a blank sheet of paper and funding was assured what alternatives to hospital would you wish to establish? How would you cater for minority mental health needs?

One of the key components in your deliberations about services ought to have been to work out with service users what they want or feel that they need.

Crisis services have become the new policy initiatives as they offer the potential of arresting a difficult situation before it becomes a full-blown emergency and escalates into a hospital admission. Your list could have included:

- crisis intervention teams;
- 24-hour crisis centres that can include short-term residential facilities;
- safe houses that offer less intensive experiences than the crisis centres;
- home treatment services where a multi-disciplinary team can support service users in their own homes;
- 24-hour telephone support;
- specialist services for people from black and minority ethnic communities.

What service users want in a crisis

Most of all what service users want is not to have any more psychiatric emergencies but if they do, they want a service that is responsive to their needs and provides a range of alternatives to hospital admission. Top of the service user list is a feeling of being in control of their own crisis. This included being involved in:

- crisis pre-planning;
- choice of treatments including complementary medicines;
- independent advocates; and
- access to quality information.

They also want to have someone to listen to them and to understand their explanation of what their crisis is about. Listening is an active process and social workers need to be skilled at this process and be prepared to spend time listening to them and not simply using the interview to detect signposts that assist with diagnosis (Golightley, 1985).

Some service users who have experienced a number of crises have developed their own checklist of what to do and what not to do when they are experiencing difficulty. This can include how to respond when they say that they do not want to take their medication when it is apparent that they are in distress. Another example is how to respond to them when they say that they are hearing voices. The point that they make is that making such a list is relatively easy when they are feeling well and upbeat but when they are distressed they recognise that they can lose their sense of what is best for them.

Intervention

The advent of the current legislations was thought to provide the means for an innovative service, which started from where the service user is rather than from what the available resources are. Thus the care co-ordinator should use their imagination to examine the best way of meeting the needs that have been identified in the assessment.

The most likely success will come from a treatment approach that will embrace a combination of anti-depressants and psycho-social support. The results of research suggest that this combination works and is more effective than either psycho-social intervention or medication on their own.[1] The psycho-social intervention could be a form of cognitive behaviour therapy; task-centred work or solution-focused work. This would be in addition to work with the more social aspects such as finances and isolation. With this in mind let us return to our case study and Mr Skeffling (Figure 5.1).

On this visual note the influencing factors have been noted. This could be taken further by the use of dotted lines where the some aspects are weaker than others or by using as above different lengths of line and point. This gives a quick and easy picture of the challenges that are facing Mr Skeffling.

---

[1] See Pritchard, 1995, p.122 for a detailed discussion of the combination of treatments.

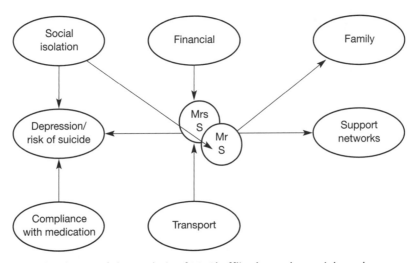

Figure 5.1: *Visual note of the analysis of Mr Skeffling's psycho-social needs*

Taking your list you could now put them into categories such as those that stabilise the situation, those that will maintain him at home, those that support the clinical input, those that bring about personal growth and enhance coping skills and those that help to improve his social interaction with his wife.

Needs or wants

One of the long running debates is the choice between what the service user may express as their want and what you and other professionals assess as their needs. Preferences may be expressed for example for a course of psychoanalysis by a service user but the cost of this is so prohibitive that it is seldom funded through the NHS. The allocation of scarce resources will always make some decisions difficult and make the realities of empowerment a challenge for social workers to meet.

Empowerment must remain the aim as well as equal opportunities and anti-oppressive practice. To practise in such a principled manner is also to work in what was called in Chapter 1 a culturally sensitive way. This is also necessary as all decisions are open to greater scrutiny since the enactment of the Human Rights Act 1998. Under s. 47(1) of the NHSCCA 1990 provision is made for the assessment of the need for community care services. This opens up the prospect of service users being unhappy with the assessment because it doesn't meet their wants as it is based on an assessment of a professional's view of their needs.

Mrs Skeffling is unhappy with the services that have been provided for her husband.

Mrs Skeffling can of course complain, as could Mr Skeffling. There is a precise complaints procedure that allows first the complaint to be resolved locally and then if that is not to her satisfaction it can move up the hierarchy. All local authorities and other care providers must show in writing how a complaint can be made. As a social worker you must inform service users and carers of their rights to complain (NHSCCA s.50). She is also entitled to her own assessment of her needs carried out in tandem with the assessment of her husband's (Johns, 2003).

You may want to consider the idea of 'spiritual healing', which has been developed by John Swinton (2001) in his interesting book *Spirituality and Mental Health Care*. Whatever your views might be about the place of spirituality it is the case that for many users and carers spirituality is a very important concept. Swinton puts forward a model of social care that includes a spiritual dimension:

> Care that takes seriously the spiritual dimensions of human beings requires an approach that draws carers into the deepest, most mysterious realms of human experience and allows them to function empathetically within a context that is often strange and alien.

(Swinton, p.136).

The question which he rightly poses is how this approach can be made accessible to people who have mental health problems. The answer if indeed there is a single answer starts with focus being placed on the people themselves rather than on the implications of their diagnosis. This requires using a different approach and asking of the service user 'What gives the service user's life meaning?' And what can be done to enhance their meaning and connectedness?

Swinton suggests that such a basic refocusing enables the professional to see the situation as the service user sees it and to accept as valid the person's concerns rather than seeing the service user as a diagnostic entity. At its best this is a developed and deep communication with the service user. This is close to my ideas of phenomenology (Chapter 2, page 23) which is a way of psychiatrists and others using empathy at the heart of their approach.

Swinton takes this on further by arguing that serious attempts to 'walk in the service user's shoes' means that we need to learn a whole new language and ideas. The term 'interpathy' has been coined to describe the entry into the world of the service user and the genuine way of attempting to understand what they are experiencing. This is more than empathy as it has the extra dimension of exploration of the service user's world.

Social workers have an important part to play in this process as one of the few professionals who can interact with the service user, their families and community. The skills that you have learned and are learning should put you in a good position to be able to help others as well as yourself to understand service users and if you choose to work in this way to help them to find spiritual meaning in their lives.

Providing for individual need

By now you should be able to see that the most effective intervention will be based upon an accurate and negotiated assessment of needs that has been agreed between the service user and the professionals. The actual provision of services will vary depending upon the individual's circumstances and the imagination of the care co-ordinator and of course the assessment of eligibility.

ACTIVITY **5.6**

Sketch out what your plan would be and check out the extent to which it meets the visual note.

My plan would be:

- To provide individual work with Mr Skeffling. This could be in the form of cognitive therapy. The aim is to help him to increase his coping skills.

- To provide information for the family about the nature of depression and suicide.

- To ensure that he has a copy of the Charter which gives him information about his rights, including the right to complain.

- To help him consider using direct payments to provide transport to the therapeutic day centre and to see the doctor. He would also like to attend a stress reduction class. To help him to enrol on the nearby history class which will also require daytime transport.

- To encourage him to go the CAB to have a financial makeover as there is a strong possibility that they are under-claiming benefits.

- To provide a short series of couple work to help them to look at their relationship and to respond to some of the anxieties and fears that Mrs Skeffling has which may be manifesting in her attitude towards him.

- To use the local MIND office to identify social support networks and to put him in touch with the local user group. They have older persons' groups and a day centre run by the members for the members. This will provide an easy route to helping Mr Skeffling to develop a network. Maintaining a network is much easier than starting one up from scratch.

- To arrange for a support worker to meet with him and go with him to the shops and get a coffee. This can also be used to encourage him to take his medication. This could be an effective use of direct payments. One of the aims is for him to develop a positive relationship whereby Mr Skeffling feels that he always has someone he can call if he needs to.

- To work with him to encourage and motivate him to want to get better and to do so by continuing to take his medication. As this has been a problem for him in the past this should be high priority.

- To work with Mr Skeffling to help him to write in a diary on a daily basis how he is feeling and what challenges he has faced. This will enable him to look back with his social worker to identify any patterns that might exist and to be able to recognise these and find ways of dealing with them.

- To develop with him a contract as the basis for future work. This will specify mutual expectations as well as what he wants people to do if it is noticed that he is becoming withdrawn or talking about it all being too much. This could also include keeping a diary record of his drinking habits.

- To arrange that he visits the 'crisis centre' and makes some contact with them. Now he is in the system he can access the services there should the need arise and there is a 24-hour help line. There is a short stay residential facility at the centre, which can be accessed through a professional referral.

Monitoring and review

Like all plans they should be regarded as work in progress and subject to modification if and when the situation dictates. The best plans are those that all parties understand and of which they have shared ownership. Mr Skeffling at present is positive and wanting to develop his coping skills and to improve his relationship with his wife. The plan can facilitate this to happen but may need to be modified as people react differently to change.

C H A P T E R   S U M M A R Y

In this chapter you have explored working with service users who need services from time to time. The emerging forms of community care, if used imaginatively and with adequate funding, should offer service users improved services. Community care assessment is crucial to this process and in this chapter the example of an older man who is depressed and potentially suicidal has been used to illustrate some of the key points that social workers must understand in order that they can play a central role in the provision of community services.

Imagination and innovation are probably not the first words most people would use to describe the process of assessment and planning but they are essential attributes that need to be a part of the overall empowering approach. Situations like the case study are often complex and to work effectively you will need to understand not just your role but how that fits in with other professionals. You will find it difficult to be empowering of others when you are unsure yourself.

FURTHER READING

Wlliams, R and Gethin Morgan, H. (eds) (1994) *Suicide Prevention: the Challenge confronted: A manual of guidance for the purchasers and providers of mental health care.* NHS Health Service Thematic Reviews. Well worth reading and contains useful checklists and discussion.

Colin Pritchard's book *Suicide – The Ultimate Rejection* contains most of what you need to learn about the psycho-social aspects of working to predict and prevent suicide. It was published in 1995 and although parts are getting a little tired it is heading towards becoming a classic read.

Useful organisations include:

Depression Alliance: www.depressionalliance.org/

MIND: www.mind.org.uk/

National Self-Harm Network: www.nshn.co.uk/

Survivors Speak Out: www.gude-informatom.org.uk

Values into Action at www.viauk.org

Mental Health Foundation: www.mentalhealth.org.uk

Chapter 6

Working with vulnerable people: adults who are long-term service users

ACHIEVING A SOCIAL WORK DEGREE

This chapter will help you to meet the following National Occupational Standards.

Key Role 1: Prepare for and work with individuals, families, carers, groups and communities to assess their needs and circumstances

- Assess needs and options to recommend a course of action.

Key Role 2: Plan, carry out, review and evaluate social work practice with individuals, families, carers, groups and communities and other professionals

- Interact with individuals, families, carers, groups and communities to achieve change and development and to improve life opportunities.
- Address behaviour which presents a risk to individuals, families, carers, groups and communities.

Key Role 6: Demonstrate professional competence in social work practice

- Research, analyse, evaluate and use current knowledge of best social work practice.
- Work within agreed standards of social work practice and ensure own professional development.

It will also introduce you to the following academic standards as set out in the subject benchmark statement that includes:

2 Defining principles

2.2.1 Social work is located within different social welfare contexts.

2.2.2 There are competing views in society at large on the nature of social work and on its place and purpose.

2.4 Social work is a moral activity that requires practitioners to make and implement difficult decisions about human situations that involve the potential for benefit or harm.

3 Knowledge, understanding and skills

3.1.1 Social work services and service users.

The nature and validity of different definitions of, and explanations for, the characteristics and circumstances of service users and the services required by them.

The relationship between agency policies, legal requirements and professional boundaries in shaping the nature of services provided in inter-disciplinary contexts and the issues associated with working across professional boundaries and within different disciplinary groups.

3.1.2 The service delivery context

The issues and trends in modern public and social policy and their relationship to contemporary practice and service delivery in social work.

The significance of legislative and legal frameworks and service delivery standards (including the nature of legal authority, the application of legislation in practice, statutory accountability and tensions between statute, policy and practice).

The current range and appropriateness of statutory, voluntary and private agencies providing community-based, day-care, residential and other services and the organisational systems inherent within these.

3.1.3 Values and ethics

The moral concepts of rights, responsibility, freedom, authority and power inherent in the practice of social workers as moral and statutory agents.

Introduction

This chapter will help you understand the type of social work that is used when working with long-term and enduring mental health service users. The example of social work with people who have a diagnosis of schizophrenia is used to illustrate various aspects that are important when engaging with long-term service users. This will help you to understand the role that social workers and other professionals play in the treatment of people with schizophrenia. Working with long-term users can be a very demanding task and brings to the fore issues about liberty, dangerousness and the different parts that we all can play in the management of mental disorder.

> *It isn't that they can't see the solution. It is that they can't see the problem.*
> G.K. Chesterton (1935)

Social work is an applied subject and:

> *... is characterised by a distinctive focus on practice in complex social situations to promote and protect individual and collective well being. At honours degree level the study of social work involves the integrated study of subject specific knowledge, skills and values and the critical application of research knowledge from the social and human sciences (and closely related domains) to inform understanding and to underpin action, reflection and evaluation.*
> (Subject benchmark statement)

Nowhere is this more relevant than in working with vulnerable people who have enduring or chronic forms of mental disorder, such as schizophrenia. This chapter will bring together some of the learning that has taken place in previous chapters about values and ethics, legal processes and context and understanding about mental disorder and some of the forms of treatment. Unlike the first four chapters in this book the last three start from the world of practice to give you the opportunity of learning about work with specific mental disorders.

Long-term users who experience schizophrenia

CASE STUDY

John is a mature student at university who lives with his father and his stepmother in an inner city area. He was admitted to the local psychiatric hospital on Saturday evening following an incident in which the police were involved. The events surrounding the admission are unclear, but it seems that John's stepmother had called the social services duty team when his behaviour became extreme and she felt threatened.

The initial contact

As a social worker you have picked up this case on Monday morning when you arrived at the office. There is a handwritten report from the duty Approved Social Worker following John's admission to hospital. It appears that he was persuaded to go into hospital on an informal basis and is there now.

Multiethnic society

ACTIVITY **6.1**

No mention has been made of whether John was from a minority ethnic group. What assumptions, if any, did you make about this? What difference would it make if John were Afro-Caribbean? Can you recall the impact of mental health in the black and minority ethnic communities?

Effective social work practice is one that is culturally sensitive, appropriate and examines personal, social and structural explanations for mental disorder. However to do this well you need to know about the different impacts that mental disorder has on people and in the case of Afro-Caribbean young men they are much more likely than their white majority equivalents to be admitted compulsorily under the MHA 1983. Figures do vary but one reliable and possibly conservative estimate is that Afro-Caribbean men are three times more likely to be admitted. Some medical practitioners suggest that stigmatisation and racism are likely to account for these differences in admission rates (Bhopal, 1998).

CASE STUDY *continued*

The next steps taken were to read John's file and to begin to refine an understanding of what had happened. The files make interesting reading and tell the story of a person who has been diagnosed as having paranoid schizophrenia and has been drifting in and out of contact with the services over the last five or so years. There is some evidence that he regularly abuses alcohol and that he likes to use recreational drugs such as cannabis and ecstasy. As a strong man he can present a rather threatening manner to people who annoy him and the previous social worker says that he has a 'short fuse'.

Assessment: the first stage

The gathering of information is an essential part of preparing for effective intervention (see Parker and Bradley, 2003). This process will probably be familiar to you and diagrammatically looks like this.

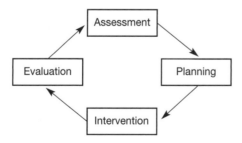

Assessment consists of a number of possibilities. In this case it could include:

- Gathering information from the user's file which helps to paint a picture of the sort of contact that has gone on with this service user and under what circumstances.

- Meeting with the stakeholders – a modernist term that includes the service user and their family or carer.

- Discussion with the other professionals who are involved with the service user.

With this in mind the case file shows that similar incidents have occurred three times over the last couple of years and John has been detained on two of those occasions. He has been in and out of employment and decided this year that he would start at university with a view to a career in the health and social care professions. John has had several social workers including a student social worker over this period and the file has some major gaps. Unfortunately the compilation of records is often treated as low priority by many social workers and it is at times like this that it becomes obvious that this means a certain degree of starting over again. When users have been detained in hospital there is a statutory requirement that a care plan should be completed and that this needs to involve the stakeholders who include John, his father and stepmother. When this has been properly carried out it will provide the full cycle of assessment, planning, intervention and evaluation for work with the service user up to the point that it is considered that the user no longer requires this level of service.

The picture that is emerging is of a young man who has few friends and remains living with his father and stepmother. He has few outside interests and the file shows that the relationships at home are not very supportive.

CASE STUDY *continued*

The visit to the home is quite illuminating as both John's father and his stepmother initially present themselves as well educated, caring people. However as the interview progresses it becomes clear that while they may be caring, they are very critical of John and his social attitude and general behaviour. His father regards it as a failure that he is unable to live up to the brother's example. He went to Cambridge University, lives and works in London and is a bright person with a lot of friends. When his father divorced and remarried John's stepmother thought that John had not got used to the idea of being in a new family and sometimes she felt his behaviour was simply to wreck her relationship with his father.

They both felt that John needed sorting out and that the services repeatedly let them down. They said that he was a danger to others when 'ill' and yet no one seemed to be interested in their view.

Dangerousness: who decides

Care in the community has had consistently bad press since the move to close down many hospitals and to relocate the service in the community. The killing in 1992 of Jonathon Zito by Christopher Clunis at a London underground station caught the public imagination and created a form of moral panic. The linking by the media of dangerousness and mental health has meant that the few incidents that have been reported have left an impression in the public mind that is difficult to erase. The effect of this has been unnecessary fear and also to put mental health professionals in the front line where any mistakes are very public.

The reality is that the thousands of decisions that are made correctly seldom get coverage. For those of you who are football fans the mental health professional is rather like the goalkeeper who makes hundreds of saves and is hardly noticed but if one error is made no one lets him/her forget. This is not to condone poor practice as this needs eradicating where it exists, but in work that is necessarily complex and involves risk management things will not always work out as you predicted.

In spite of the above it is important that we study the cases where things have gone wrong and make sure that we learn from them. Subsequent inquiries have been well reported and in general show a degree of what is called 'system failure' characterised by a breakdown in communication and understanding between the various agencies that are involved. This has in turn resulted in a lack of trust not only by the public in services, but also it seems by government ministers who seem to be ever more influenced by interest groups as well as the impact of adverse publicity. However, this degree of panic reaction has and is being conducted largely in a research vacuum. The reality is that we simply do not know if the public is at an increased level of risk from mentally disordered patients (Coid, 1996).

CASE STUDY

In 2003, 19-year-old Daniel Rogerson was convicted of manslaughter with diminished responsibility after attacking and stabbing to death a 78-year-old neighbour in a sleepy village in Lancashire. In another instance Paul Kahn attacked and killed a complete stranger called Brian Dodd on a North Wales beach. Both of the attackers were people who were known to the services and had a history of severe mental illness. Both had a history of carers having sought help from services and in their opinions they were not responded to in an appropriate way.

However the evidence that is available shows that although the incidences are in reality very low, there are a small number of people who are likely to engage in violent acts. It is evident that people with severe mental disorder who exhibit violent behaviour are much more likely to kill themselves rather than others.

The ability to predict who will carry out such acts is limited and far from a science. With this in mind Coid calls for:

- better training for mental health professionals in assessment and treatment;

- more effective training in risk assessment and management; and

- patients who behave dangerously and default from treatment should not be allowed to become ill in the community.

(Coid, p.967).

In John's case there was concern about his behaviour, but there was no evidence that he was actually violent. It is important to distinguish between what is verifiable evidence and what is speculation. Among the factors that need to be considered are:

- past history of violence which is the most reliable means of determining future conduct;

- poor compliance with treatment and aftercare;

- substance misuse; and

- recent severe stress.

This stage is still about gathering information about John and trying to determine what this episode means for him and his family. Once you have got about as much information as you are going to get, the next step is to determine what to do with the information.

Involving service users in risk assessment and management

Research commissioned by the Joseph Rowntree Foundation examined the involvement of users in their own risk assessment and management. The work was carried out in England and interviews were in-depth with users, carers and professionals. The findings include:

> *Many service users were aware that they could pose a risk to other people when experiencing psychosis and wanted to reduce the chances of this happening. Levels of agreement between service users and professionals about risk and how to respond to it ranged from full agreement to very little or none; and serious gaps were sometimes found in information held about service users that potentially put themselves and others at risk.*
> (Joseph Rowntree Foundation, April 2004)

This shows that there is a lack of consistency in the overall approach to working with risk and risk management and much depends upon the individual professional. The researchers suggest that there needs to be a format for assessing risk and the subsequent management plan incorporates service users' views (Langan and Lindow, 2004).

The hospital visit

Shortly after the family has been interviewed John is visited on the ward. An initial and brief conversation with the nurse in charge reveals that John is in quite a distressed state and is receiving anti-psychotic medications. He is hearing voices and can exhibit challenging behaviour from time to time. The initial diagnosis has been confirmed as paranoid schizophrenia. This is also an important time for you to discuss with the nurse your safety when meeting with John. It is not the time for bravado as putting yourself in a potentially dangerous position is good for neither you nor John. In this instance the view is that the situation is safe, but as a precaution you are given a waist fitting alarm.

Understanding the impact of schizophrenia

In Chapter 2 some of the characteristics of schizophrenia were described which is information that you would need to know prior to your visit with John to enable you to discuss the treatment and care plan for John with the other professionals. The model that was used in this chapter suggests that even with disorders that have a physiological or genetic component to them stress plays an important part. People with schizophrenia have a high sensitivity to stressful events which can trigger the onset of an episode of schizophrenia. Such events can be located in life events such as divorce or loss of someone close to them, but could also include the loss of work or other events outside of their personal or family domain.

One of the features of some forms of schizophrenia is the experience of auditory hallucinations, commonly known as 'hearing voices'. Some people who have schizophrenia also have feelings of thoughts being inserted into their mind or have visual hallucinations. Interestingly these are usually culturally specific with people in the west hearing voices from space or computers while people from less developed countries may report hearing voices that are more to do with religion or demonic possession.

ACTIVITY 6.2

Understanding what the arrival of schizophrenia must mean to people is crucial for you as a social worker. We talk about walking in the other person's shoes and you should find whatever source you can in order to do this. You may be fortunate in that on your course there are service users who have had mental health experiences and they might be willing to share these experiences with you.

Understanding visual hallucinations is a feature of the movie A Beautiful Mind *that shows the life of the brilliant professor John Nash who works at an Ivy League University in the USA and has been a lifetime sufferer from schizophrenia that includes visual hallucinations. If possible try to see this film.*

CASE STUDY *continued*

During your interview with John he begins to act rather distanced and when you check with him he tells you that he is hearing voices. This poses a real challenge because you have never come across this before and you are not sure what to do.

Working with people who are hearing voices and experiencing delusions

Katie Glover (2000) has written a very practical guide for communicating with people who have mental health problems and there are some other guides that will help you to understand the best way of working with people who experience delusions or hallucinations.

There are some very practical steps including:

- Recognition that the service user is experiencing voices instead of ignoring them and trying to carry on as if nothing was happening: 'Are you having difficulty following what I am saying?' 'Are you hearing voices?'

- Acknowledge the difficulty and distress that are caused by hearing voices: 'It must be very hard for you to continue with this conversation, thank you for sticking with it.' (Glover, 2000, p.157)

If John has said that it is very distressing you need to acknowledge that you understand and then be prepared to wait for a while or to postpone your interview. What you do not do is be dismissive of John's voices. They are real for him and you are starting from where he is.

Some people experience delusions which means that they are confused about who they are or often where they are. This can be disturbing for the family and disconcerting even for professionals. By and large the work that you would do with people who are deluded is simply a mixture of empathy and honesty. Consequently, faced with someone who says that they are from the secret service you might suggest, 'But now you are in this hospital and I want to work out with you how we can best help you.' This approach acknowledges the presence of the 'delusion' but avoids collusion with it and tries to establish a foothold in reality.

Hospitalisation

John is in hospital on an informal basis which means he can discharge himself at any time, subject to the holding power that is Section 5, MHA 1983, which gives nurses and doctors the right, in certain clearly defined circumstances, to keep John on the ward until a doctor can reassess his condition and evaluate the risks to John or to others (Chapter 3 covers this aspect). He is on an acute admission ward that specialises in the assessment of a patient's disorder and attempts to discharge as soon as possible. John is known to the services, consequently the assessment will not be to determine if he has schizophrenia, but to try to stabilise his current situation to the point where John can return home and a community treatment plan can be agreed between the stakeholders.

As we have seen in Chapter 3 informal patients can refuse treatment in line with common law. This right to refuse can be mediated if the patient is assessed as not having the capacity to make such decisions. Questions around capacity or lack of capacity are ones that medical practitioners have to address, often consulting with other professionals.

John is reasonably content to take his medication which the RMO has prescribed and which includes anti-psychotic medication. This follows, you have learnt, a typical pattern for John. He will take his medication when in hospital and for a short while after discharge back to the community but he then stops his medication or becomes erratic in his self-administration. Changing this into a more reliable pattern becomes one of the goals for his treatment in the community.

CASE STUDY *continued*

John has responded well to treatment and after ten days is already being considered for the next step of returning to the community. You have made more visits to the family and to John on the hospital ward.

If John had been detained on a section of the Mental Health Act 1983 the staff would be obliged to ensure that John was given specific information as soon as practicable about his admission and other information including rights about treatment, detention, renewal and discharge (s.132). This is considered to be good practice and similar information should be made available to John as an informal patient.

Life on the ward is a return to the familiar for John, but even so his experiences have not been overwhelmingly positive. This fits with evaluations of many service users who report concerns about:

- feelings of being unsafe on the ward;

- lack of meaningful activities to keep them occupied;

- insufficient information about their disorder and expectations of the ward staff;

- low levels of one-to-one interaction with the professional staff; and

- lack of involvement with planning their treatment and return to the community.

(See DoH *Mental Health Implementation Guide*, 2002)

Many service users report the importance to them of one or two individuals with whom they had made a significant relationship or the importance of the other service users who helped them to get through the difficulties that they were in. But others feel that they were largely ignored and saw the RMO insufficiently for it to be a major factor in their recovery.

Substance abuse has also emerged as a problem on many acute admissions wards. Staff have to be vigilant to prevent the use of recreational drugs such as crack cocaine on the ward. This not only confuses the treatment regime of patients but can have an impact on the life of the ward in general and other patients in particular. Dual diagnosis is the term used to describe the coexistence of mental disorder with another diagnosis. This can be mental disorder and learning disability or mental disorder and substance abuse. In some inner city areas as many as three patients in ten have a dual diagnosis involving substance abuse with the consequence that they spend longer in hospital than do single diagnosis patients and are up to four times more likely to commit acts of violence than those with the single diagnosis of schizophrenia (*Rethink Sane*, Zito Trust, 2003).

These challenges pose real problems for hospital staff and striking the balance between the need for formal observation, and vigilance against drug dealers can result in a mass of rules and procedures, the net effect of which can make living on a ward more like being in a custodial institution rather than a hospital. Service users need to be listened to and engaged wherever possible in the running of the ward and their care.

Planning for successful intervention: working across agencies

The Care Programme Approach (CPA) has meant that the planning for John's discharge has already got underway and an initial plan has been developed in conjunction with John and using information from the family. This is put alongside the diagnosis, the previous notes and the views of the medical practitioner and the nursing team.

Working across agencies and between professionals from different disciplines has long presented a challenge for professionals who are trying to deliver a community based service that is effective. The introduction by the government of the National Service Framework and the Care Programme Approach (CPA) in 1991 were just two of the features of the new modernised mental health service. The government had a clear idea that the CPA would be the system that ensures that service users would be supported in the community and that this would reduce the chance of them drifting out of contact with the services. The CPA should produce a holistic service that is co-ordinated and uses a key worker or care coordinator system that takes the lead in all aspects of the involvement with the service user (more detail is provided in Chapter 3).

One of the key aspects of this is an assumed common vision of how the service might work. In one study all the professionals thought that they had clear objectives and a commitment to involving service users. Central to this is the attitude of the workers who are involved and the few evaluations of this tend to show that among nurses, social workers and support workers there is a shared view and a desire to change practices to be more user-focused (Carpenter et al., 2003). However implementation of these modernised services across the country is patchy and research carried out by the NHS Executive and the Social Services Inspectorate in 1997 confirmed that a seamless service that was user-focused and not resource driven, was still an ideal in many parts of the country that was waiting to be implemented (Bartlett and Sandlands, 2003).

The introduction of the National Service Framework (NSFMH) in 1999 set out seven specific standards for providers of services to meet and these included a range of services from community outreach to secure hospitals. The standards apply across the board to both health and social service providers, and standards four and five refer explicitly to inter-agency work and the importance of multi-disciplinary assessment. There is also enabling legislation in the form of the Health Act 1999 that enables local authorities and health authorities to transfer funds to each other in order to promote a seamless service and to generally improve the quality of the service.

When teams come together this creates a common approach, but it would be a mistake to think that this means that everyone has an equal say. In particular, according to anecdotal evidence, doctors and psychiatrists, are ostensibly happy to be a part of the multi-disciplinary team, but only when they retain, to use an American football analogy, the quarterback position (the star position). When this is put alongside research it shows, not surprisingly, the acquiescence of the service user to medical practitioners. Low (2004) writes that what is missing is the concept of active interest and involvement of lay people or, in our terms, service users. The effect of this is to create a new hierarchy in which the service user still remains at the bottom, the professionals, other than doctors, are in agreement with each other while doctors are still on top.

Service users on top

It was the recognition that service users needed to be at the centre of reforms that led the government to embark on a comprehensive listening process to enable the service user voice to be heard. The listening exercise, 'Your health, your care, your say', allowed the public to speak directly to ministers, health professionals, and each other on how improvements could be made to their local services. Included in the 143,000 contributions were many mental health service users and carers. This exercise resulted in July 2005 in the publication of a new White Paper.

The White Paper: *Our health, our care, our say: a new direction for community services*

This Paper recognises how NHS and social care services work together and how these services could adapt to provide individuals with the health and social care services they need closer to their homes The White Paper, *Our health, our care, our say: a new direction for community services*, aims to:

- *change the way these services are provided in communities and make them as flexible as possible;*

- *provide a more personal service that is tailored to the specific health or social care needs of individuals ;*

- *give patients and service users more control over the treatment they receive;*

- *work with health and social care professionals and services to get the most appropriate treatment or care for their needs.*

(DoH *White Paper: Our health, our care, our say: a new direction for community services*, January, 2006)

To achieve these aims will require that all agencies learn to work better together and that service users and carers will have more say in the type of service that they wish for and need. This will give greater emphasis to ideas of partnership – something that training and educational courses will need to remember.

To keep up fully with all the changes that are being proposed there is no better place than to go to the DoH website and to click onto the White Paper Bulletin www.doh.gov.uk/ ourhealthourcareoursay

As far as John is concerned you are lucky to be working for one of the newly formed community mental health teams, and it is in this context that you are trying to plan with John a course of treatment and care that will help him to stabilise while in the hospital and eventually to make the important move into the community. Assertive Outreach teams are something of a new invention and in reality it is too early to pass judgement about their effectiveness.

ACTIVITY 6.3

Think about the realities of working together in one multi-disciplinary team and the notion that service users and workers are in acquiescence to medical practitioners. Is this a good thing? To what extent do you think that this is inevitable? What impact will this have on you if you are to work in a multi-disciplinary team?

Even after recovery from an acute phase, most patients struggle to reintegrate into the community. In John's case, there were few community links prior to hospitalisation so the task of reintegration is even more difficult. Where home life is difficult the importance of work and outside activities increases and part of your task may be to identify what is available in the community. This could include sheltered workshops, day centres, hostel or user groups. A good supportive environment is often to be found at voluntary organisations like MIND, the mental health charity, or other active mental health groups.

Had John been detained on a treatment order (s.37,s.3 etc.) there is a duty on primary care trusts or health authorities and social services departments to provide, in co-operation with the voluntary and independent sector, aftercare services until they are satisfied that the user no longer needs this service. This has caused some local problems as the duty is placed on the area which the user goes to on discharge. This has resulted in some arguments between authorities as to who is responsible and a ruling from the High Court that it is the area from which the patient came when admitted that bears the financial responsibility, with the exception of people who are of no fixed abode (Bartlett and Sandland, 2003).

ACTIVITY **6.4**

If John lived in your area what resources would be available for him? It would be helpful to you if you could spend a little time looking around at just what is available. If you have a local MIND *shop they usually have a list of the resources that are in your area and sometimes community mental health teams have similar information.*

Early intervention

The frequent contact with services interspersed with periods of low or no contact is sometimes also referred to as the 'revolving door' and presents a challenge to services. These patterns seem to be entrenched for John, which is unfortunate as research suggests that a key determinant in a person's career as a mental health patient is the speedy and effective response to the initial episode (Frangou and Bryne, 2000).

The first episode, like it was in John's case, happens usually in the late teenage years or early twenties and probably like John the behaviour can go undetected for several months or even longer. This is largely because of the contextual factors that include:

- erratic behaviour that is also a characteristic of late teenage years;
- the known use of recreational drugs like cannabis which confuse the symptoms of psychosis;
- the first signs may be negative ones such as withdrawal, social isolation, and emotional flattening, none of which on their own may cause significant concern; and
- people who hear voices are often reluctant to tell people of this partly because they feel that people will think of them as being mad!

Trigger events

The model used in Chapter 2 helps to conceptualise about the onset and some of the factors that can result in mental disorder such as schizophrenia. Whether the occurrence of an episode is as a result of some event which effectively triggers this, or whether it is inside the person is unclear. However the likelihood is that it is as a result of key events that produce considerable stress for the user.

With the above in mind can you speculate what the triggers might be in John's case? Think of those that might be personal for John and those that are more social.

Trigger events could be the result of some 'unresolved' issue for John, which has left him conflicted; this might be something hugely significant like emotional or other abuse whilst growing up. It could also be as a result of a stressful event that he has been unable to resolve, this could be starting at university and not being able to make social contacts, exacerbated by living at home. It might also be a combination of these.

Although the lifetime prevalence of schizophrenia is about 1% which may seem low to you, the impact of schizophrenia brings with it huge social and personal costs. People who are diagnosed with this severe disorder literally join another tribe and can become isolated. The impact of the disability can be understood in the same way that Oliver (1996) writes about the social model of disability. The disorder itself can have a significant impact upon the person and their families but this is magnified by the association in the public's mind with dangerousness and the difficulties that the public has in dealing with unusual and unpredictable behaviour.

Consequently it really is in everyone's interest that early recognition is made and an appropriate response is made. The use of medication in the first episode is reported as being more likely to succeed as in the initial phase the user may be more responsive to treatment (Frangou and Bryne, 2000). This can take the edge off the psychotic symptoms and be an effective maintenance tool but on its own is probably insufficient.

The prognosis for people diagnosed with schizophrenia is that about 80% will recover but over 70% will have a second episode within a five to seven year period (Frangou and Bryne, 2000). This suggests that treatment should be considered longer term than the initial episode and that long-term courses of antipsychotic medication may be advised. However the most likely successful recovery or maintenance is to be found when the medication is a part of the overall treatment plan and a more holistic approach is used. This fits in with the model that was covered in Chapter 2 that brought together the different components that may impact on and lead to a mental disorder such as schizophrenia.

Although the dominant paradigm is medical the evidence that supports the primacy of a uni-directional approach is hard to find. As a social worker you need to guard against this approach being the only one that you will work with as it brings with it some consequences for the service user and can make your role a secondary one. The advantages of using a more holistic assessment and modelling approach are that you can begin to understand why more Afro-Caribbean young men are diagnosed with schizophrenia than their equivalent white male counterparts. It also helps you to understand the role that families can play in the onset of schizophrenia and, importantly, in the treatment.

Intervention

It is generally considered that family circumstances are important determinants of future success or relapse with people who have schizophrenia. The research shows that relapse is more likely for users who have a diagnosis of schizophrenia if, after a period of hospitalisation, they return to a family that is overly critical or is emotionally over involved and controlling (Brown, in Butler and Pritchard, 1983, p.90). This resulted in the development of a concept called **expressed emotion** (EE), and the rather surprising finding that users may fare better in the community if they do not return to their families.

More recently Pharoah, Mari and Steiner (2000) conducted an evaluation of the effectiveness of family interventions for people with schizophrenia in line with the drive towards increasing the evidence base for various interventions. This evaluation took Brown's work as the starting point for their evaluation and has produced strong evidence that confirmed their work. Even so the use of this approach in a practice setting is limited and it has by and large been left to one or two researchers to 'promote' this approach. The work of Leff, Kuipers and Lam (2002) is an example of this approach being slowly spread to other practitioners (nurses and social workers) through the Thorn Initiative.[1]

Expressed emotion is a clinical concept and the presence of high expressed emotion has a high predictive value. EE is actually a research technique and measures things like critical comments, hostility and over involvement that in turn produce emotions of various strengths. Experiencing high EE can cause considerable stress for some people and, it seems, especially for people with schizophrenia. Work with families involves trying to get families to move from expressing the negative side of emotions to developing techniques and mechanisms that demonstrate the positive aspect of emotion.

Measuring expressed emotion can be carried out using a standardised assessment schedule using the Camberwell Family Interview (CFI) that was developed in the 1960s. This is usually completed by the user's family and because the person has been admitted to hospital the completion of the schedule occurs soon thereafter. Interviews are usually taped and then subject to analysis or scoring over three dimensions which are:

- **criticism** which is measured by scoring the number of overtly critical and specific comments that have been made;

- **hostility** which is scored when there is rejection of the patient as a person or a combination of general criticism and rejection;

- **over involvement** which includes exaggerated emotional responses, usually self-sacrifice and overly devoted behaviour, over protection that is inappropriate to the patient's age, and difficulties in maintaining boundaries.

This requires practice and training as the tone and content of the interview are also taken as measures of the expressed emotion.

---

[1] The Thorn Initiative is an extensive course in psycho-education approaches pioneered by the Maudsley NHS Trust and the University of Manchester

The treatment model as expressed by Leff et al. (2002) is underpinned by a view that can be summarised as follows:

- schizophrenia has a biological basis but people who are diagnosed are particularly sensitive to stressful events which makes them vulnerable to relapse;

- family members need to join in with therapeutic work as they are both affected by the arrival of schizophrenia and may have contributed unwittingly to the relapse and possible onset;

- honesty, openness and clear communication are important in order to share information about the nature of the disorder and to recognise the limitations of this knowledge;

- families have positive as well as negative features and it is important to build on the strengths; and

- this form of work needs to be carried out together with other forms of intervention and supervision.

As you can see, this is, in reality, a psycho-social education form of intervention in which your role as a social worker is to play the role of educator with the family. While social workers need to be aware of the medical side of mental disorder it is important that they retain their own skill base and capacity to work in an empowering way. This approach is empowering as the family is encouraged to learn more about schizophrenia and to work with the therapists to determine their own solutions to the problems as they see them.

Evidence is being gathered from other countries which shows similar results to that achieved in the UK. Kalfi and Torabi (1996) carried out a study in Iran that included a cross-cultural comparison. This revealed that expressed emotion is an important factor in predicting relapse among users who have schizophrenia who lived in Iran. In a similar vein studies about the impact of high EE in families that contain a user with bipolar disorder or unipolar disorder also look promising.

While to become fully competent in this type of intervention does require additional training the general principles of these approaches can be usefully applied to many situations. As a social worker you could be the champion of an approach that is empowering of the service user while retaining the treatment ethos of a uni-directional approach. This approach encapsulates social factors such as unemployment, substance misuse, poor social networks, and high expressed emotions and puts them alongside the diagnosis of mental disorder as equal partners rather than as subsidiary parts (Tew, 2002).

Working with John and his parents in a holistic manner puts them centre stage and offers them the opportunity to learn about schizophrenia and to understand the effect that their communication patterns may have upon John. In some cases it may be advisable for John to leave his parents' home and to live in other accommodation and 'manage' his relationship with his parents in this way. This enables him to escape the 'trapping' patterns of communication but also does not place the blame for his disorder on the parents. After all, it is very unlikely that parents consciously choose to relate to their children in ways that create problems.

Caring for the carers

Carers of people with long-term mental health use may find the process challenging and debilitating. Those carers who provide regular and substantial care for a person on CPA are covered by Standard Six of the National Service Framework, which to be met, would mean that they receive their own written care plan following discussions with them and your assessment of their physical and mental health needs. This needs to be carried out annually at least.

Assertive Outreach

Assertive Outreach teams are a part of the reform to mental health services in the community. They work in an intensive manner with long-term users of mental health services who are considered to be difficult to engage in treatment. John would probably fall into this category given his history of non-compliance with medication and his readmissions to hospital.

The Sainsbury Centre, in 2003, reviewed the people skills that are needed to work with the typical service user who receives Assertive Outreach. They came up with a list of personal and professional attributes that included being able to:

- work with service users in informal settings;

- work with service users and families in an accepting and certainly uncritical manner;

- hold realistic expectations of service users and the scope for complete recovery; and

- relate to service users' experiences of mental health, possibly through their own experience of oppression or of mental health.

    (Sainsbury Centre, 1998)

The same document also describes some of the evidence that underpins the assertive outreach approach and claims that they can reach a large percentage of hard-to-engage service users and that they are generally liked by service users and their carers. When these teams work well they provide an integrated service that consists of a variety of professional groups including community psychiatric nurses and social workers.

ACTIVITY 6.6

Make some enquiries, if you do not already know, whether there is an Assertive Outreach team in the area in which you live. If they do exist get their information for service users which should help you to understand more about this specialised multi-disciplinary service.

The plan

Your work with John will be informed by your own understanding of the challenges that he faces and your assessment of the trigger events. This is nearly always achieving a balance between what the service user wants, what you and other professionals think that the service user needs and the reality of what is actually available. The process should begin early and have the service user at the front of the deliberations about treatment options. The CPA assumes that the care plan will be drawn tighter with the active involvement of the service user and that they will have agreed and signed the action plan.

ACTIVITY 6.7

With John the plan could take on a number of different shapes and at this point with the little information that you have you should make some notes of three possible plans.

Your three plans would of course be drawn up following discussion with other professionals, John and his family. They might include (but not be limited to) these.

Plan one

Do nothing and let John leave hospital and return home taking antipsychotic medication. They have your telephone number and if the situation worsens they can contact you. The justification for this is that it's the least invasive plan and of course uses the least direct resources. This assumes that you have all decided that John is not a risk to either himself or to others.

Plan two

John returns home taking antipsychotic medication, and with the offer of family work to reduce the level of expressed emotion in the family and with your support he will eventually return to university.

Plan three

John moves to supported living accommodation in town, his family are offered ten sessions to help them to understand how they can change some of their behaviours to help his recovery, he starts going to the local MIND day centre and takes part in a support group run by service users for people hearing voices. The local Assertive Outreach team offers him a package of comprehensive services including monitoring his medication.

C H A P T E R   S U M M A R Y

Several themes should be evident in this chapter, not least of which is working in partnership with service users. Because of the debilitating nature of schizophrenia and the low level of public knowledge about the condition you will have to move at a slow pace and be acting as both a therapist and a psycho-social educator. The use of a holistic assessment and psycho-social methods of working is likely to be the most effective social work intervention with people who have long-term schizophrenia (like John).

As a social worker you have a crucial role to play in holistic assessment and in order to fulfil this role you need to be a professionally competent worker who has sufficient knowledge to be able to hold your own with medical practitioners without unnecessary acquiescence to them. Your work should be characterised by empowerment and a high level of specific knowledge about the resources that you have available in your area and about what works.

Priebe and Slade's (2002) book *Evidence in Mental Health Care* (Hove: Brunner-Routledge) has some very useful chapters about what works and with whom. See the chapter on the user perspective about what counts as evidence.

For help and advice about benefits consult *The Big Book of Benefits and Mental Health* from Neath Mind, 32 Victoria Gardens, Neath, SA11 3BH. A ten-page proforma is available online from www.rightsnet.orguk/pdfs/AA

Subject benchmark statements are best accessed through the Quality Assurance Agency (QAA) website: www.QAA.ac.uk and then into subject benchmarks.

Joseph Rowntree Foundation, York: www.jrf.org.uk

Chapter 7
Working across organisational and professional boundaries

The current range and appropriateness of statutory, voluntary and private agencies providing community-based, day-care, residential and other services and the organisational systems inherent within these.

3.1.3 Values and ethics

The moral concepts of rights, responsibility, freedom, authority and power inherent in the practice of social workers as moral and statutory agents.

3.1.4 Social work theory

Research-based concepts and critical explanations for social work theory.

The characteristics of practice in a range of community-based and organisational settings including group care within statutory, voluntary and private sectors.

Introduction

Sunlight is the most powerful of disinfectants and electric light the best policeman.
Mr Justice Brandis (1914)

This final chapter brings together some of the themes from earlier chapters under the heading of working together to provide an integrated service that is efficient and effective. Providing an integrated service that will protect children is used as an example although the need to work together applies across the whole range of services. The links with other chapters, such as Chapter 4 on child and adolescent services, will be all too apparent but in this chapter the primary focus is upon providing the service user with a needs-led service that does not involve them having to be referred to other agencies.

Children are rightly the focus of this chapter because they may be in need of mental health services because of individual mental disorder; they may be being parented by someone who is themselves experiencing mental disorder or they could be the unfortunate subject of a fabricated mental disorder. In the UK 2–5% of children are brought by their carers to the attention of Primary Care Teams with mental health issues as the main presenting problem. It is likely that many more children with mental health problems do not present at all (Spender et al., 2001).

At the extreme end the pressing issue of child protection and mental health is explored using the Victoria Climbié Inquiry and others as examples of the need to put children first, irrespective of different professional boundaries. The Green Paper *Every Child Matters* (September, 2003) focuses on the support that parents and carers should have; early intervention and effective protection; issues of accountability and integration regionally and nationally and the need for workforce reform.

Every Child Matters: Next steps was published in March 2004 and set out the ways in which the proposals in the Green Paper could be enacted. At the same time legislation was introduced in the form of the Children Act 2004 to set out a new national service framework for children whilst retaining the 1989 Children Act.

Community-based services have now become one of the dominant organisational forms from which mental health services are provided and this chapter will help students to understand the roles that they can perform in such services. These will include working as a 'care co-ordinator' to provide direct services and as an 'assessment officer' to determine the extent that services should and can be provided.

Evidence-based practice is introduced to point you to the ways that the professions will progress.

Working with service users as individuals and with service user action groups has become a standard way of working but one that requires considerable skill and understanding, both of which are explored as an aid to student learning.

Service users' views

A more recent development of these ideas is termed 'The Circle of Involvement ' which is a simple way of understanding how it is necessary and what steps need to be taken to ensure that service users become more involved. This was conceived out of work that was carried out in the Trent region and brings together key components such as education and training, government policies, service development and workforce development. By visualising these components as a circle that is seamless and that one component feeds in to the other it is possible to work towards greater involvement at any stage (*Principles for Practice*, December 2005).

Involving service users owes its origins to the Children Act and the 1990 NHS and Community Care Act, both of which placed the involvement of service users on the agenda. The idea of citizen participation goes back much further than this and can be traced to town planning and the work of Sheri Arnstein (1969) who first developed a 'ladder of participation' and subsequently to the community social work and community development movements of the 1970s. This has gained considerable momentum with the requirement put onto social work courses to involve service users in all aspects of social work training. Where this is taken seriously it will undoubtedly be a transformatory process and could result in major changes to education and training. However it is still too early to evaluate if the involvement of service users will be more than just a fine idea.

The mental health service user movement includes those that are involved at the governmental level such as MIND and YoungMinds, both of which regularly submit high quality detailed analyses to inform policy making. There are also examples of patient controlled services such as Camden Mind and the influential Patient Councils. In addition there are local user groups which may be affiliated to the national bodies such as SANE or MIND or Survivors Speak Out and specialist groups such as Women in Special Hospitals.

Service users of course need to be consulted about the services that they receive to help find out what sort of intervention works well and why. However, in contrast with clinical drugs trials, all too often the evaluations that have been carried out are about satisfaction with the services received when what is desperately needed is an evaluation of what worked and the extent to which it worked.

Service users can be involved at different levels:

• individual level where they work with the professionals to determine what is the most appropriate way of responding to their mental health needs;

• group level with service users working together, with or without professional facilitation, to support each other;

- activist groups where they comment upon aspects of service delivery and challenge or inform conventional operational practices;

- involvement at a strategic level to plan services or training courses such as service user groups or as individual representatives;

- involvement in national bodies to campaign for changes and to offer government policy-makers advice and assistance.

The involvement of service users varies according to what level they want to become involved at and what is available. At each level there is also the prospect that within that level will be specialist interests such as black and minority ethnic or women's groups. The key for social workers is to form alliances with service user groups and to work with them in ways that will recognise the contribution that both can make in moving towards a mental health service that is user-focused and emanicipatory.

ACTIVITY 7.1

Some organisations work as pressure groups campaigning for what they see as necessary changes to mental health law and services. Now is the time for you to go onto the internet and check out at least one of these sites. The YoungMinds website www.youngminds.org.uk is usually one of the best for a wide range of coverage of mental health issues.

The involvement of adult service users has been slow to get underway and at times somewhat tokenistic. However there has been progress with even less children and adolescent involvement. It is surprising given the legislation about children's rights that they can be so easily overlooked and the adult view of what children want dominates. Even the present proposals to reform the legislation state that when considering individual treatment for children and young people the clinical team must consider the wishes and feelings of the child while they must take *'proper account'* of the parental view. This took into account the view that children may not be competent to determine their own treatment but this is seemingly contradictory with the Richardson Committee suggestion that children should be considered competent from the age of 10 –12 and that competence should be assessed according to the Gillick judgement.

ACTIVITY 7.2

What reasons can you come up with to explain why the perspectives of children and young people have not been considered in respect of mental health services? How valid is this? Would lowering the age at which people can vote to 16 make any difference?

The Equality Act 2006

The Equality Act received Royal Assent on 16 February 2006. This legislation will bring about some major changes and may well provide impetus to the greater involvement of people with mental health problems in mainstream service delivery. The first part of the Act effectively sets up a replacement body for the Equal Opportunities Commission (EOC), the Commission for Racial Equality (CRE), and Disability Rights Commission (DRC). The new body is to be called the Commission for Equality and Human Rights (CEHR) and will promote equality irrespective of age, religious belief, gender, and sexual orientation and will come into being October 2007. The second part of the Act will extend protection against discrimination and provide protection for people against discrimination on the grounds that they have no religious belief.

Working towards an integrated service

The idea of working together to provide a seamless service to service users is far from new. In 1976 as a part of a research team we published my first major piece of mental health research (Jones et al., 1985). This was a project led by Professor Kathleen Jones of York University and was a tracer study to examine the destinations of nearly 200 patients who had been discharged from York psychiatric hospitals over a two-year period. In that research we examined the ways that agencies tried to work together or to be more frank the ways that they didn't manage to work together! Back then we talked about agencies 'collaborating' a rather strange term given that collaboration means working with the enemy! Since then I have followed with personal and professional interest how things have moved on and it is timely to revisit the idea about working together.

Integrated services are services that are joined together to provide one access route for service users. Such services imply common training to at least some extent and shared values. Multi-disciplinary approaches retain the professional and often organisational identity of the professional involved.

Multi-disciplinary teams

The multi-disciplinary team exists both as a community mental health team, and in a form that includes professionals who work in the team part-time and also work back in their own agencies. A child mental health team could comprise members as in Figure 7.1, although this will vary from agency to agency. The first point for involvement will usually be a referral from the family doctor to this team for assessment, and if intervention is planned a care co-ordinator will be appointed who will carry the responsibility for the case. This can be the scene for some power struggles between the professions and also within the professions. General practitioners are often more comfortable dealing with another medical colleague than relating to a different professional. Consultants will point out that they have clinical responsibility for the individual and hence medical–legal responsibility. This has been further compounded with the emergence of nurse prescribers. These issues can be sorted out and it is important that the multi-disciplinary team establishes clear operating procedures.

Figure 7.1 *Child mental health team*

The emergence of a new, planned workforce

The National Workforce Action Team was established to determine what the demand for staff might be and what type of staff was needed for the modernised mental health service. Poor workforce planning has resulted in much of the present services developing in an ad hoc way that reflects more circumstance, history and influence than effective planning. The slowness of establishing joint planning teams has hindered the development of widespread effective integrated services. The Workforce Action Team pointed out that poor planning was in part the result of the limited links that agencies had with each other and the general lack of enthusiasm across professions to implement flexible working practices and cooperation (Alcock, 2003).

One of the exciting developments in community mental health has been to recognise the importance of factors such as community support and networking. This is important work, which can make a huge difference to the experience of the service user. This has coincided with the emergence of a new support worker with a new type of qualification. These roles are close to those of social work but are more limited in their scope. Some professionals see this new form of worker as a threat to their role and simply a means by which government can cut the wage bill. What do you think?

The management of mental health professionals

Careful risk assessment is necessary for any person who is engaged in direct work with people who are under the age of 18 years and are provided with health or social care services, especially in the light of the Allitt Inquiry (see later in this chapter). This includes health screening to ensure that they are fit for employment and that any condition which is revealed can be managed in a way that will not adversely affect their work with service users or colleagues. This is a balancing act that requires careful assessment, especially in the light of the need to reduce discrimination that people with disabilities, including mental disorder, experience.

The list of Inquiries that permeate social work makes monumental reading but there are valuable lessons that must be learnt if the profession is to progress and vulnerable people be better served. It is to these that we briefly turn.

Learning from Inquiries

Two Inquiries are described, the most recent concerning the circumstances around the death of Victoria Climbié and the other that of the nurse Beverley Allitt who was convicted of the murder of several children at the hospital ward where she worked. They are but two of many, far too many, Inquiries into the untimely death of people who in different ways had expected the services to have done more to protect them. Although each Inquiry has some specific lessons that need to be learned, together they point out that some of the basics that make up competent practice have not been taken on board.

The Victoria Climbié case

Victoria was a healthy, lively, happy young girl who had been sent to England by her mother in the hope that she would be well educated and achieve her potential. What parent would not want this for their child? However this was not to be and in the space of a few months she was tortured, humiliated and in the end died. At the post-mortem examination she had over 128 separate injuries all over her body. In the final few weeks of her life social workers made attempts to see Victoria but made the incorrect assumption that she and her carer had moved. That the result was tragic is self-evident but that it could have been prevented is a shocking indictment of professional services including social workers (Johns, 2003).

Were Victoria's carers mentally disordered or just sadistic people? There certainly is an argument that can be made to support the view that anyone who tortures and kills a person must be mentally disordered even though in this case the sentencing suggests that this was not an argument that found favour with the jury.

What lessons can be learned?

1. Social workers and other professionals should learn to listen to children and not to dismiss what they say. This needs to be put alongside observations that add to the child's explanation.

2. Social workers should be clear about the purpose of contact with service users and what information needs to be gathered to clarify levels of accountability (recommendation 5, Climbié).

3. Staffing levels, training and management all are in need of improvement and monitoring.

4. As far as mental health services are concerned the following has emerged:

   - more support for young carers is needed;
   - the overall approach should be multi-disciplinary with a lead professional involved; and
   - there should be a common assessment framework.

The Child and Adolescent Services (CAMHS) received additional funding to develop a more comprehensive approach to child mental health problems (see Chapter 4). In addition to these measures the various bodies charged with monitoring compliance with national standards are asking social services and trusts to provide information about the arrangements for safeguarding children and to ensure that their staff are suitably trained and aware of their responsibilities towards children.

Example of Sure Start work: Parenting Matters

Parenting Matters is a course that is run in numerous parts of the country. It is a 30-hour programme held over 12 days to help parents share experiences, remember their own childhood, develop listening skills and learn how to set clear boundaries. Early evaluation shows increases in self-esteem and reduction in authoritarian attitudes. (Parenting Plus; Sure Start, 2004)

The Allitt Inquiry

In the early part of 1991 three children died suddenly and unexpectedly on the children's ward at Grantham and Kesteven General Hospital. There were further 'emergencies' later that year which finally aroused suspicion and a police investigation started. The suspicion was that someone was deliberately harming children on the ward. Eventually this was traced to a young nurse called Beverley Allitt who was subsequently charged with four murders, nine attempted murders and nine accounts of causing grievous bodily harm. While on duty in the children's ward in her local hospital, she tried to kill at least 23 children by injecting them with insulin and potassium, choking, breaking ribs and asphyxiation.

Beverley Allitt suffered from the rare Munchausen's Syndrome by Proxy which is a variation of Munchausen's Syndrome, in which individuals fake symptoms or harm themselves so that they can be the centre of attention. The syndrome is named after a German soldier renowned for telling exaggerated stories. There is still no convincing theory about the causes of this disorder and it is quite rare. Beverly Allitt was sentenced to 13 life sentences and was transferred to a high security psychiatric unit.

Sir Cecil Clothier conducted the Inquiry that followed in 1994. Among many findings was the following comment:

> *Taken in isolation, these fragments of medical evidence were not all very significant nor was the failure to recognise some of them very culpable. But collectively they would have amounted to an unmistakable portrait of malevolence. The principal failure of those concerned lay in not collecting together those pieces of evidence.*
> (Clothier, 1994, p.131)

There are concerns that over-vigilance may result in spurious identification of false risk, a topic which resulted in widespread discussion, including in the House of Lords where the possibility of such a condition being widespread was considered and the possibility of false diagnosis discussed (Lords Hansard, 1997).

> *Put at its simplest, there is all the difference in the world between a Beverley Allitt, whose severe personality disorder led her to murder young children, and a mother who invents reasons why she and her child should visit the doctor. Yet under the all-embracing banner of MSBP, and in the hands of the untrained, the two are treated as being practically indistinguishable. It does not matter whether one calls the condition MSBP or factitious illness by proxy, or by any other name. The point remains the same.*
> (Lords Hansard, 1997)

What lessons can be learned?

The Allitt Inquiry demonstrated four aspects that are particularly relevant for this chapter:

- The need to look out for patterns that help to explain what otherwise might look to be phenomena that are unconnected. This means keeping an open mind and discussing your ideas with others.

- The need to establish and operate a strong whistleblowing protocol that allows other professionals to raise concerns about questionable practice and for these to be followed up.

- The importance of staff screening, and regular supervision and monitoring of performance.

- The professional culture should be underpinned by values and driven by the empowering practice that is open to challenge.

In light of these Inquiries we need to ask ourselves just how we protect children who are at risk and promote their positive mental health and ability to cope with adverse and stressful situations.

Child protection

The policy and legal context

The main legislation is the Children Act 1989 which applies to a person under the age of 18 and the Mental Health Act 1983. Various provisions in the Children Act permit the psychiatric examination of a child although once the child is of sufficient understanding, using the Gillick rules, the child can refuse to be examined (Eldergill, 1997). If the court decides that there is a chance of significant harm a Child Assessment Order (s.43 Children Act 1989) can be made that authorises a child assessment including a psychiatric assessment. There are additional powers available to the courts that include the making of an interim care order and care order. Harm includes impairment of health, which includes mental health (s.31 (9) Children Act 1989). This is important as the community care legislation in general does not apply to children or only applies in a qualified way. (For a more detailed explanation of the relevant law in this area see Chapters 3 and 4 in Robert John's *Using the Law in Social Work*, 2005, in this series).

It is important to realise that although considerable attention goes to the relatively small number of children who are at risk of being or who have actually been seriously abused, a much greater number of children have their development seriously challenged by adverse events, many of which are outside of their control or influence. These need to be considered by social workers and others.

In 1998 the government published a Green Paper called *Supporting Families*, which made clear that the government's mission was 'to put children first'. This was an important statement at a time in the UK when the divorce and separation rate is rising and children can be the innocent victims of these separations. The changed circumstances of parents can mean reduced income levels, changes to school, meeting new 'step-parents' and much more. The policy is to support parents and children undergoing these changes through a wide variety of initiatives.

The publication in 2003 of another Green Paper *Every Child Matters*, which followed the tragic death of Victoria Climbié, called for the strengthening of existing services to provide a universal and non-stigmatising service that children and young people could access through the education system, as well as the creation of new and more focused services for those children who needed additional support.

New duties were imposed on local authorities and what is termed their relevant partners under section 10 of the Children Act 2004. This is an enabling piece of legislation designed to be a key driver in the Government plans to provide more comprehensive service for children. Included in these is the duty on local authorities and partners to co-operate to improve children's well being.

Well-being is defined in the five outcomes for children to:

- Be healthy
- Be safe
- Enjoy and achieve
- Make a positive contribution and
- Achieve economic well being.

The speed of the changes is fast and the extent of the impact probably little appreciated by those who are not directly involved. Fortunately the relevant website permits close and detailed scrutiny and some free downloads of key documents is permitted.

One of the changes will be how services are organised and key to these is the establishment in most areas of Children's Trust that will take the lead role in the coordination of local health, social care and education services as well as other agencies such as Sure Start that may be working with children. This raises all sorts of issues about governance and even in some areas issues about geographical boundaries. The majority of areas will have had to have a Children's and Young People's Plan in operation by April 2006 which will set out in an accessible format the strategic direction the area will take to safeguard children.

The workforce capacity to respond to this initiative is crucial and we know that large numbers of people who work with children are presently unqualified and most likely underskilled (DoH Core Standards, 2004).

This is a high level of integration, which will mean many agencies will have to rethink how they can engage in collaborative processes. Among the children who have been identified as requiring a high degree of integrated services are those who have 'special circumstances' which includes looked after children; children of parents who experience mental health problems and children who are exposed to domestic violence and family breakdown.

One of the key parts of the new integrated service has been the design and trialing of what is known as the Common Assessment Framework (CAF). This is a standardised approach to the assessment of a young person's needs and should provide early indication of the requirement for services. This is an holistic assessment that includes the role of parents, carers and the impact of external factors such as environment. As this is such a cornerstone of *Every Child Matters* most areas have seen a comprehensive rollout programme being established. All forms are available on the web and are in downloadable word format so you can familiarise yourself with this assessment tool (www.everychildmatters.gov.uk/resources-and-practice).

So far we have examined Inquiries to learn about when things go wrong and how the government is making a huge investment that should promote children and young people's life chances.

Does the separation of parents adversely affect the mental health of their children?

It is estimated that at least one in three children will experience parental separation before they reach the age of 16. Should this trend continue this would need to be looked on as the norm for families and we need to recognise that children need to learn coping skills that will better equip them to cope with these transitions. The research commissioned by JRF shows that no matter how well handled these separations might be they are difficult for children and young people to cope with. Although most will experience this as a period of unhappiness and distress that they work through, there are others who will struggle to cope with the effects that this has had on their lives. A small minority will experience mental health problems and some will need specialist help. In *Foundations* (2004) *Together and Apart* the JRF research shows among other highlights that the following are relevant:

- the quality of the parental relationship is important for the child's successful adjustment to post-separation circumstances;

- the older the child the more difficult it is to adjust to being in a stepfamily;

- extended families can play an important supportive role at the time of separation;

- at the time of separation the child's interests can be overlooked as a consequence of the preoccupation of the parental need;

- different children want different services, some like these to be at school and others want services that are outside of school.

However children whose parents separate can benefit from the separation if it is handled well and it is much healthier to grow up in a reconstituted family that is at peace with each other than to remain in a family whose parents are continually at war with each other.

ACTIVITY 7.3

The Connexions service is one of the new developments that have brought together services like youth work and careers guidance but they also offer much more. Spend some time either on the internet or visiting the local Connexions office to find out the range of facilities that they can either offer or co-ordinate. www.connexions.gov.uk

---

Connexions have developed differently in different areas but you should have found that they offer a one-stop high street drop-in facility. Personal advisors are often located in local schools and again can provide career guidance as well as personal and group counselling. This can provide a stigma-free valuable support service for young people as well as an early warning of problems. They refer young people on to other professions when it is clear to them that the person's needs are greater than they can provide for.

Problems that occur in the first few years

The risk of depression in mothers after childbirth (postpartum period) is greater than at any other time, with at least one woman in ten having a depressive episode within 12 months and the risk is greatest in the first three months after childbirth (Spender et al., 2001). Depression among adults has been covered in earlier chapters and we need to consider the impact on the child where the mother is distracted from the usual childrearing to deal with her own problems.

The cause of depression in mothers most likely has a biological component to it as does having a history of mental disorder, but once again social factors such as isolation, unemployment, lack of a confiding relationship, lack of supporting social networks are all factors that are likely to increase the risk of depression occurring. Childbirth is a major life event, mostly full of joy but also an event that requires a considerable change in lifestyle of the parent(s).

The impact on a mother and partner, if there is one, can be considerable and signs that would usually be picked up as possible indicators of depression can often be dismissed as simply the impact of a new baby. Depression needs to be distinguished from the onset of 'baby blues', which is very common and usually occurs in the first ten days but then goes, and depression, the onset of which is much later. There are numerous scales, such as the Edinburgh Postnatal Screening Depression Scale, that can be used to assess for depression. Health visitors and general practitioners should always be alert to this possibility, not least of which is being aware of the risk to the child in this situation.

RESEARCH EXAMPLE

In a programme developed with the Sainsbury Centre for Mental Health in Edinburgh, Staffordshire and Lewisham health visitors were trained to use a post-natal questionnaire and problem-solving skills. The impact of this training was evaluated using random control trials and the results suggest that the intervention was at least as effective as the use of anti-depressant medication (Sure Start, 2004).

Sure Start projects

We can get a good look at where government policy is going with the Sure Start pro-gramme that aims to rectify some of the consequences of social exclusion and inequalities and in so doing to achieve better outcomes for children, parents and communities by:

• increasing the availability of childcare for all children;

• improving health, education and emotional development for young children;

• supporting parents as parents and in their aspirations towards employment.

There are now 524 Sure Start projects across the country both in inner city and rural areas and the government is aiming to open 1,700 centres by 2008. The centres have been introduced to help tackle child poverty by improving children's social and educational development and helping parents balance work and family life. They are trying in locally determined ways to work in disadvantaged areas to influence service delivery as well as to provide direct services themselves. The work is evaluated both at local and national level and early indications are positive that these projects are making a difference.

While adult community health teams focus almost exclusively on the effect on the adult of severe and enduring mental illness, Sure Start programmes focus on depression in adults, mainly mothers, and the effect this had on their children's emotional development. The involvement of Sure Start programmes in the CAMHS programmes also varied, often dependent on the networks and background of the co-ordinator. Some projects had CAMHS workers seconded to them on a part-term basis, others were used to provide the 'user perspective'. What most of the Sure Start projects wanted was to help bring about changes in mental health services to move away from a reactive clinic style approach to a more proactive community-based style of working. Services need to be accessible and at the same time offer privacy and confidentiality (YoungMinds, Sure Start, Conference 2003).

The innovative approach used by Sure Start to develop positive mental health is seen by them as integral to their overall approach. They have targeted key factors for intervention and influence and have created very attractive placement and work settings for social workers. Sure Start have established crèches, parent circles and parent education groups, all of which have the effect of helping develop awareness of the importance of promoting resilience and emotional health among parents and children. There is a long way to go but the impact of these initiatives ought to be significant in the long term.

Problems that occur in school age children

There are numerous behavioural problems that might beset some school age children. One of the difficult tasks is being able to differentiate between what in the present day is con-sidered to be unruly or unusual behaviour and when that becomes a source of genuine concern as an indication of mental disorder. Not least of these is the somewhat controver-sial presence of attention deficit hyperactive disorder covered in Chapter 4.

Children whose parents have mental disorders

The effect on children who have at least one parent with a mental disorder is worthy of consideration. If we go back to the importance of stress as an intervening variable it is possible to realise the impact that mental disorder of a parent can have on the child caught in this situation. A study of 100 reviews of child deaths where abuse and neglect were factors showed that parental mental disorder was present in one third of these cases (*Red Manual Code of Practice*, 2004).

Research carried out in the Netherlands examined the available literature and gathered together a panel of mental health practitioners all of whom had direct practice experience of working with children and their families (Rikken, 1995). They sought to identify what needed to be present to promote positive mental health. Out of this research came a number of findings including:

- the seriousness and chronicity of the parent's disorder was a significant factor;
- the quality of the relationship between the parent with mental disorder and the remaining parent was significant;
- the age and resilience of the child was an important variable; and
- the nature and extent of the social network to support the family.

The intervention in the Dutch project centred on work with the child and the 'healthy' parent, work to educate the family about the nature of the disorder and the development of social support networks. This is supported by other research showing that community-orientated and proactive initiatives are delivering measurable improvements in parenting skills (Davis and Spur, 1998; Hutchings et al., 1998; Walker, 2003).

Chapter 2 pulled together various factors that put people at risk of developing mental disorder. The impact on the children whose parents have mental disorder was described as being: problems at school, isolation and lack of specific information about their parent's mental disorder and prognosis. The outcome for children whose parent has a mental disorder will vary according to the severity of some of the variables mentioned earlier and will also depend upon the resilience and coping abilities of the child. However if a child grows up in a household where one of their parents has a chronic mental disorder they are at a greater risk of developing mental health problems than if their parent did not have a mental disorder.

This is considered to be so important that YoungMinds have suggested to the government that whenever an adult is diagnosed as experiencing a mental disorder, the law should require that the psychiatrist determines if that adult has parental responsibility for a child and if so that the psychiatrist has a duty to inform social services. This would allow extra support to be given to the family and child to mitigate against some of the negative factors surrounding their parent's mental disorder.

Of course there are other factors that can seriously disturb child development, such as having carers who abuse drugs, something that is becoming more and more common.

Safeguarding children in whom illness is fabricated or induced

A Department of Health Guidance document for Area Child Protection Committees recognised that children may be at risk as a result of their carer attempting to have them diagnosed with some form of illness. Here we see played out a familiar tension referred to by the earlier information from the Lords Hansard about how to protect children from real but rare events, while not wrongly accusing carers of deliberate attempts to harm the children in their care.

There are four main ways that the carer may fabricate or induce illness in a child. These include:

- signs and symptoms;
- falsification of medical records;
- falsification of bodily fluids and/or letters or records; and
- induction of illness by different means.

(adapted from DoH, 2001)

It is important to realise that while as a social worker you should be aware of this phenomenon and alert when vulnerable people are at risk, the diagnosis of this disorder needs to be left with specialists who are experienced and have training in this type of diagnosis.

Understanding children

Sally Gorin at the NSPCC has carried out a literature review that draws together evidence about how children have experienced living with domestic violence, parental substance abuse and parental ill health, both physical and mental. This can make some children very vulnerable and in need of support. The themes that emerged included:

- children are much more aware of their parent's problems than the parents imagined which in turn can lead to high levels of concern about their parent's safety;
- children tend to use informal support and talk to either parents, siblings or friends;
- when they did go to professionals they were not always satisfied with their contact and felt that they were not listened to, whereas what they wanted was someone to listen to them and in whom they could place their trust;
- age-appropriate information was needed to help children to understand what is going on in their family.

(Adapted from Gorin in *Findings,* 2004 JRF)

The following gives a good picture of what the experience must be like and how children feel.

> *Sadness and isolation that children may experience can be perpetuated by the stigma and secrecy that surrounds domestic violence, parental substance misuse and ill health. Some children report feeling depressed, having problems making or maintaining friends, having a disrupted education or experiencing bullying.*
> (*Findings*, May 2004, p.2)

147

Not all children suffer long-term effects and they are often very resilient and bounce back from these adverse conditions.

Assessment of risk and resilience

It is commonly thought that when children are exposed to adverse and stressful situations their mental health will suffer. This is in spite of evidence that suggests that there is not a causal relationship. Clearly in a relatively small number of instances children are at immediate risk of serious harm and the numerous Inquiries where this was overlooked make sobering reading. However it is also the case that many, many more children experience turmoil and adversity in their lives and not only survive it but actually do well. Is it possible that in concentrating upon the individual risk, for all the right reasons, we might overlook the positive effect that social factors might make to help the individuals cope with adversity? Have we got the balance right between protecting children from risk and promoting in them the ability to bounce back when they experience difficulties? Certain key factors crop up time and time again when we look at how some people experience distress and cope. These are described by the term resilience.

Resilience has a near-universal meaning to it and is best summed up as:

> *Resilient children are better equipped to resist stress and adversity, cope with change and uncertainty, and to recover faster and more completely from traumatic events or episodes.* (Newman and Blackburn, 2001, p.1)

There is extensive documentation of both risk and resilience in the social science and social work literature (Rutter, 1999; Walker, 2003) and the common factors that can be deduced fit well into the schematic chart that was presented in Chapter 2. If we take the main headings used in the chart we can list the following factors.

Social causation factors
- Having a strong extended family;
- successful schooling;
- network of friends
- having a role outside of the family – volunteering, sports, clubs;
- member of a religious community.

Psychological factors
- Warm, supportive carers;
- good parent–child relationships;
- parental harmony;
- confiding relationship with at least one parent.

Personal

- Age;

- higher IQ;

- social skills;

- humour;

- temperament.

(Adapted from Newman and Blackburn, 2002)

However where the above are not present and replaced by low income/poverty, over-involved parents and social exclusion then the child's ability to bounce back from adverse and stressful events is much less likely to occur. Although as social workers we are often involved in short-term crisis resolution, the most damaging impact on child development is most likely to be where the situation is chronic and with little prospect of improvement.

A psycho-social educational approach with parents

ACTIVITY **7.4**

What strategies could be adopted in order to help children to cope better and develop resilience? Write down what you think could be done and by whom. Spend a few minutes on this task.

It ought to help if you refer to Figure 2.1 that was used in Chapter 2. This will give you direct clues about where the need might be but this tool is better at analysis rather than strategy. What works for children coping with adverse situations is having the support of their extended family, neighbours or mentors and having close friends in whom to confide, rather than the specific activities of professionals. (Newman and Blackburn, 2002). How different was this to your ideas? Should the social work task be one of mobilising community support, supporting, befriending and building up a data base for service users to make contact with each other? Children need to have opportunities to learn coping skills in the face of difficult situations. They need to develop self-esteem and to feel valued if not at home then outside of the home. Social workers and others should always look to the strengths as well as the problems in each individual's situation.

Empowering intervention

The psycho-social model of intervention provides a conceptual tool for social workers to work with the diverse populations that make up the UK.

ACTIVITY 7.5

As a social worker working with Asian children you realise that they are trying to respond to their parents' cultural practices when at home and to the cultural norms of their white friends when at school. As they are getting older the tension between the two is becoming more apparent and their behaviour at school is becoming a problem. The teachers at the local school have asked you to give some advice to them. What would be your response?

Of course there is no easy answer. The use of the psychosocial model allows you to conceptualise some of the problems and to see them as potentially having an adverse impact on the children's development. You are trying to work anti-oppressively but just who is your client? What cultural norms would you respect?

Evidence-based practice

How do we know what works, why it works and with whom it works best? These questions should be at the heart of the reflective practitioner and throughout this book an attempt has been made to locate practice alongside evidence. If social work is to stand alongside other professions we must be able to support our claim with evidence that what we do actually works.

There are a number of information systems that provide up-to-date research reports about mental health and other work with service users. Facilities such as the Cochrane Library, The NHS Centre for Reviews and Dissemination and the newly created Social Care Institute for Excellence (SCIE) will provide academics and practitioners with electronic forms of data and research evaluations. But this on its own it is insufficient and social workers will need to take advantage of the new social work curriculum to enhance their own evaluative and research skills in order to make best practice common practice.

C H A P T E R   S U M M A R Y

This chapter has drawn together the idea of working together to provide the kind of effective mental health service that service users want and that will provide children with protection. Social workers can be involved as members of a team that responds to the needs of users including children. Children need to be more involved not just with their care and treatment but also should be consulted about service design and delivery. That they are not says more about our lack of imagination and faith than their abilities.

Child protection can never be far away from social work discourse and two Inquiries were considered to demonstrate what happens when things go wrong. Children also need to be recognised as potentially strong and resilient and the social work role might well be to enhance these strengths rather than concentrate on weaknesses. It is a reality that many children experience trauma and loss and work through this transition and emerge relatively unscathed.

Using the psychosocial model of intervention, various ways of working with parents were addressed and the advantage of this to social workers is that it allows us to make full use of a holistic view of mental disorder.

FURTHER READING

Clothier, C. (1994) The Allitt Inquiry considered the Beverly Allitt case, answering such questions as how she was allowed to qualify as a nurse, why her crimes were not detected sooner and what can be done to prevent another similar tragedy occurring in the future? The Inquiry also makes recommendations for changes in procedures.

Tony Newman and Sarah Blackburn (2002) of Barnardo's Policy, Research and Influencing Unit have produced a must-read paper that provides an in-depth examination of many of the issues raised in this chapter. It is called Transitions in the Lives of Children and Young People: Resilience Factors, published by the Scottish Executive Education Department and available electronically. www.scotland.gov.uk/publications

Quentin Spender et al. (2001) *Child Mental Health in Primary Care.* Abingdon: Radcliffe Medical Press is an excellent text that covers numerous child mental health problems and more. Includes check-lists and assessment questionnaires.

Every Child Matters sets out for consultation a framework for improving outcomes for all children and their families, to protect them, to promote their wellbeing and to support all children to develop their full potenial. DfES (2003) *Every Child Matters: The Next Steps* and *Every Child Matters: What You Said* (2004) Nottingham: DfES. Can be accessed at www.dfes.gov.uk/everychildmatters/

The booklet *Principles for Practice* (contains the Circle of Involvement ideas and more can be obtained from the Trent Multi Professional Deanery by emailing Rachel.Hawley@tsha.nhs.uk

WEBSITES

Useful contacts

www.nhsdirect.nhs.uk

www.mind.org.uk

www.sane.org.uk

www.nsf.org.uk

www.doh.gov.uk/mentalhealth

www.bbc.co.uk/health/mental/

MACA (Mental Aftercare Association)
maca.bs@maca.org.uk
www.maca.org.uk

Parenting Plus
www.parentlineplus.org.uk

Winston's Wish
info@winstonswish.org.uk
www.winstonswish.org.uk

Social Care Institute for Excellence
www.scie.org.uk

Young Minds
enquiries@youngminds.org.uk
www.youngminds.org.uk

Lords Hansard
www.publication.parliament.uk

All JRF Findings are published on their website: www.jrf.org.uk

Glossary

Approved doctor under s.12 of the 1983 Mental Health Act A s.12 doctor is approved by the Secretary of State as *'having special experience in the diagnosis and treatment of mental disorder'*. Each region has its own selection panel, which sets standards for doctors who seek approval in their area.

Approved Social Worker (ASW) A qualified social worker who has undergone a 12-week additional training course. In order to comply with the 1983 Mental Health Act and ensure their independence, the ASW must be appointed and employed by the Local Social Services Department.

Behaviour modification Based on the idea of learning theory and conditioning. Intervention focuses on the relearning of behaviour.

BNF Stands for the **British National Formulary** reference text, which is published twice a year and contains up-to-date information about the maximum dosage of medication for patients. Hospital wards should always have the latest copy available.

Bolam test Where a healthcare professional is not considered to be negligent if s/he adopts the practice which a responsible body of professionals (e.g. psychiatrists, nurses or social workers) accept as appropriate.

CAMHS Child and Adolescent Mental Health Services.

CMHT Community Mental Health Team.

Cognitive therapy A treatment intervention, available on the NHS, that focuses on mal-adaptive patterns of thinking that affect the person's behaviour.

Commission for Social Care and Inspection and the Commission for Health, Audit and Inspection 2004 The National Care Standards Commission (NCSC) was the body that oversaw the commitment to health and social care standards in the independent sector, as set out in the **Care Standards Act (2000)**. The NCSC was established in April 2000 and abolished in April 2004 under the **Health and Social Care (Community Health and Standards) Act 2003 (HSCA)**.

The main body of the NCSC was merged with the Social Services Inspectorate **(SSI)** to form the **Commission for Social Care and Inspection.** The Private and Voluntary Healthcare Directorate (the department responsible for regulating all independent hospitals in England) combined with the Commission for Health Improvement and part of the Audit Commission to form **The Commission for Health, Audit and Inspection (CHAI)**. CHAI is now formally referred to as **The Healthcare Commission**.

Court of Protection Part VII of the 1983 Mental Health Act aims to protect the property and financial affairs of an individual who is incapable of acting because of a mental disorder. The MHA also provides safeguards for anyone authorised by the Court of Protection (Court) to manage the patient's finances.

CPN Community psychiatric nurses are qualified and experienced psychiatric nurses who play a major role in the supervision and treatment of patients in the community. Along with ASWs, psychiatrists and others, they have a pivotal role in community mental health and outreach teams.

CSIP NIMHE (National Institute of Mental Health for England) has now been absorbed into a successor body Care Services Improvement Partnership (CSIP). CSIP embraces eight programmes. They are the National Child and Adolescent Mental Health Services (CAMHS) Support Service; Health in Criminal Jusitice; the Integrated Care Network; Integrating Community Equipment and Support; the National Institute for Mental Health in England; the Health and Social Care Change Agent Team; the Valuing People Support Team; and Children for Change. It has an annual budget of more than £30 million. Chief executive: Richard Humphries. Website: www.csip.org.uk

Diagnosis Forms part of the assessment process and the identification of specific mental disorder in which reference is made to either the **DSM IV** or to the **ICD–10** reference texts both of which classify mental disorder.

Expressed emotion This term is used usually in the sense that the family may have 'high expressed emotion' that is having a adverse effect on the service user. This includes over-involved parents and a highly critical atmosphere.

Family therapy The focus is on working with the family to restore the family system to a more functioning unit.

Home Office Mental Health Unit The Mental Health Unit was formerly known as C3 Division and it exercises the Home Secretary's powers in respect of restricted patients under the 1983 MHA.

HSC Health service circular.

HSG Health service guidance.

LA Local authority.

LAC Local Authority Circular.

Mental Health Act (MHA) 1983 Although this legislation is over 20 years old it is still the primary legislation in this area. It is primarily about the compulsory admission, treatment and discharge of people who are diagnosed as having a mental disorder.

Mental Health Act Commission (MHAC) The Mental Health Act Commission (MHAC) is a Special Health Authority within the NHS. Commissioners are appointed by the Department of Health for a period to undertake this statutory role. The MHAC oversees the operation in respect of detained patients (see s.120 and s.121). The MHAC publishes a Biennial Report and a number of guidance notes on the interpretation of the various parts of the Act. Commissioners regularly visit all hospitals in England and Wales and meet with detained patients. Based on current information, it is envisaged at the current time that the MHAC will be merged with the Healthcare Commission (CHAI).

Mental Health Act (MHA) hospital managers For the purposes of the 1983 Mental Health Act (MHA) it is important to differentiate between 'MHA managers' and any other hospital staff who may also be referred to as 'managers' in terms of a general management structure, e.g. a directorate manager or CMHT manager is not the 'MHA manager' in respect of the MHA. It is the 'MHA managers' who are the formal detaining authority under the Act, not the registered medical practitioner/responsible medical officer (RMO). At common law, 'the managers/NHS Trust' … are legally liable for any deprivation of liberty which is not justified by the Act.

Mental Health Act (MHA) Hospital Managers' Review Patients who are detained in hospital may request that the reasons for their continued detention in hospital are reviewed by the MHA hospital managers. The MHA hospital managers (s.23) can order the discharge of an unrestricted detained patient.

Mental Health Review Tribunal (MHRT) The Mental Health Review Tribunal (MHRT) is a court governed by the Lord Chancellor's Department. The purpose of the MHRT is to hear the patient's appeal against detention and reception into guardianship or supervised discharge can be made (see Part V of the MHA). The MHRT comprises three people: a legal member, lay member and medical member. The MHRT can order the discharge of a patient with or without conditions.

Nearest relative (NR) Clearly defined under s.26 of the MHA 1983.The nearest relative (NR) is usually, but not always, the patient's next-of-kin. Section 26 explains how to identify the NR. A common mnemonic is '**How Should Folk Be Graded, Give Us NewS**'. That is, **h**usband/wife; **s**on/daughter; **f**ather/mother; **b**rother/sister; **g**rand–parents; **g**randchild; **u**ncle/aunt; **n**ephew/niece; **s**ame sex partner. If the relatives are of equal standing, the eldest is preferred. In-laws are usually excluded. The patient cannot choose who the NR should be.

National Institute for Clinical Excellence (NICE) Conducts research and evaluations of various treatments and publishes guidance and advice.

National Institute of Mental Health England (NIMHE) See Care Services Improvement Partnership (CSIP).

PGO The Public Guardianship Office which is the executive agency based in the Lord Chancellor's office and which carries out the work of the Court of Protection.

NHS National Health Service.

Patient The term used throughout the MHA as is the male pronoun. Social workers use the term service user, implying more of a partnership exists between themselves and the 'user' of the service but patient is still used in the hospital setting.

The Mental Health Act 1983 provides that, unless otherwise stated and except in relation to the Court of Protection, the word *patient* means 'a person suffering or appearing to suffer from a mental disorder' (s.145(1)). In the context of tribunal proceedings, the patient is simply the person whose case is under review. There are a number of different types of patients, e.g. informal patients , voluntary patients and restricted patients.

PHCT Primary health care team.

Prognosis The medical assessment of the future course of events and probable outcome of the patient's mental disorder.

Psychoanalysis Based on Freud the aim is through the client/therapist relationship to resolve conflicted states of mind. Not available on the NHS.

Responsible medical officer (RMO) The psychiatrist who has full clinical and legal responsibility for a patient detained under the 1983 Mental Health Act. Described within the 1983 MHA as the doctor who is in charge of the treatment of the patient. They will usually be a consultant psychiatrist and approved under s.12 of the MHA as having a special experience in the diagnosis and treatment of mental disorder.

Second opinion appointed doctor (SOAD) A registered medical practitioner (experienced psychiatrist) appointed by the MHAC to provide an independent opinion in respect of Consent to Treatment under Part IV of the 1983 Mental Health Act.

Section 12 approved doctor Approved by the Secretary of State as '... *having special experience in the diagnosis and treatment of mental disorder*'. Each strategic health authority/region has its own selection panel which sets standards for doctors who seek approval in their area, receives and scrutinises applications and grants approval under the 1983 MHA where appropriate.

SHA special health authority.

SSD Social services department.

Statutory A requirement dictated by Act of Parliament, e.g. the 1983 Mental Health Act.

Statutory duty A duty that must be complied with if contained within an Act of Parliament.

Statutory instrument Relates to delegated legislation drafted by the relevant department under powers attributed by an Act of Parliament. Statutory regulations are most commonly drafted as Statutory instruments and laid before Parliament, e.g. The Mental Health (Hospital, Guardianship and Consent to Treatment) Regulations 1983.

References

Ahmed, B. (1991) *Interpreters in Public Services* (eds Baker, P., Hussain, Z. and Saunders, J.). Birmingham: Venture Press.

Alcock, J. (2003) *Mental Health Services – Workforce design and development – best practice guidance*. London: DoH.

American Psychiatric Association (1994) *Diagnostic and Statistical Manual of Mental Disorders (DSM–IV)*. Washington DC: American Psychiatric Association.

Arnstein, S. (1969) A ladder of citizen participation in the USA. *Journal of the American Institute of Planners*, Vol 35, no 4.

Banks, S. (2002) *Ethics and Values in Social Work*. Basingstoke: Macmillan.

Bartlett, P. and Sandland, R. (2003) *Mental Health Law, Policy and Practice*. Oxford: Oxford University Press.

Bean, P. (1986) *Mental Disorder and Legal Control*. Cambridge: Cambridge University Press.

Bhopal, R. Spectre of racism in health and health care: lessons from history and the United States. *British Medical Journal*, 27 June 1998; 316: 1970–1973.

Blackburn, D. and Golightley, M. (2004) European Sociological Conference paper. University of Lincoln.

Bowers, L., Clark, N. and Callaghan, P. (2003). Multidisciplinary reflections on assessment for compulsory admission: the views of Approved Social Workers, general practitioners, ambulance crews, police, community psychiatric nurses and psychiatrists. *British Journal of Social Work*, Vol. 33,961–8.

Brammer, A. (2003) *Social Work Law*. Harlow: Pearson Educational.

Brock, A. and Griffiths, C. (2003) *Trends in the Mortality of Young Adults Aged 15–44 in England and Wales 1961–2001*. Office of National Statistics: Health Statistics Quarterly. See also website: www.statistics.gov.uk

Brown, G.W. and Harris, T.O. (1978) *The Social Origins of Depression*. London: Tavistock.

Butler, A. and Pritchard, C. (1983) *Social Work and Mental Illness*. Basingstoke: Macmillan.

Campbell (1999) *Training for Mental Health 3: Exploring key areas*. Brighton: Pavilion Publishing.

Campbell, J. in K. O'Hagan (ed) *Competence in Social Work Practice: A practical guide for professionals*. London: Routledge, Kegan Paul.

Carpenter, J., Schneider, J., Brandon, T. and Wooff, D. (2003) Working in multidisciplinary mental health teams: the impact on social workers and health professionals of integrated mental health care. *British Journal of Social Work*, 33, 1081–103.

Clark, C. (2000) *Social Work Ethics*. Basingstoke: Macmillan.

Clothier, C. (1994) *Report of the Inquiry into Beverley Allit: The Allit Inquiry* (1991). London: HMSO.

Cochrane, R. (1983) *The Social Creation of Mental Illness*. London: Longman Applied Psychology.

Coid, J.W. (1996) Dangerous patients with mental illness; increased risks warrant new policies, adequate resources, and appropriate legislation. *British Medical Journal* 312: 965–6.

Crawford, K. and Walker, J. (2003) *Social Work and Human Development*. Exeter: Learning Matters.

Cree, V. (2002) The changing nature of social work in R. Adams et al. (eds) *Social Work: Themes, issues and critical debates*. Basingstoke: Palgrave.

Curran, C. and Bingley, W. (2003) Seclusion: Part 1 3, *Openmind*, Nov/Dec, No 124, p.29.

Curran, C. and Grimshaw, C. (1996) Supervised discharge. *Openmind* Sept/Oct, No 81, p.28.

Curran, C. and Grimshaw, C. (1998) The use of Guardianship under the 1983 Mental Health Act. *Openmind*, Sept/Oct, No 93, p.24.

Curran, C. and Grimshaw, C. (2000) Advocacy in mental health. *Openmind*, Jan/Feb, No 101, p.24.

Curran, C. and Grimshaw, C. (2000) Consent to treatment for medication under the 1983 Mental Health Act. *Openmind*, March/April, No 102, pp.24–5.

Curran, C. and Grimshaw, C. (2000) Mental Health Review Tribunals. *Openmind*, May/June, No 103, p.24.

Curran, C. and Grimshaw, C. (2000) The Mental Health Unit at the Home Office. *Openmind*, July/Aug, No 104, p.24.

Curran, C. and Grimshaw, C. (2000) Review of treatment under s.61 of the Mental Health Act 1983. *Openmind*, Sept/Oct, No 105, p.24.

Curran, C. and Grimshaw, C. (2000) Review of treatment under s.61 of the Mental Health Act 1983 revised. *Openmind*, Nov/Dec, No 106, p.24.

Curran, C. and Grimshaw, C. (2001) Police holding power under s.136 of the 1983 Mental Health Act. *Openmind*, Jan/Feb, No 107, p.24.

Curran, C. and Grimshaw, C. (2001) Leave of absence under s.17 of the 1983 Mental Health Act. *Openmind*, Nov/Dec, No 112, p.24.

Curran, C. and Grimshaw. C. (2002) Compulsory admission to an NHS or independent hospital, *Openmind*, Jan/Feb, No113, p.29.

Curran, C. and Grimshaw. C. (2002) Information for patients detained under the 1983 Mental Health Act. *Openmind*, Jan/Feb No 119, p.29.

Curran, C. and Grimshaw. C. (2002) The Role of the RMO under the 1983 Mental Health Act. *Openmind*, July/Aug, No 116, p.29.

Curran, C. and Grimshaw. C. (2002) The Court of Protection patients. *Openmind*, Sept/Oct No 117, p.29.

Curran, C. and Grimshaw. C. (2002) Doctors approved under s.12 of the 1983 Mental Health Act. *Openmind*, Nov/Dec No 118, p.29.

Curran, C. and Grimshaw, C. (2003) Detention of patients under Part III of the 1983 Mental Health Act. *Openmind*, March/April No 120, p.29.

Curran, C. and Grimshaw, C. (2003) Warrant to search and remove patients under s.135 of the 1983 Mental Health Act. *Openmind*, July/Aug No 122, p.29.

Curran, C. and Grimshaw, C. (2004) Seclusion part 2. *Openmind*, March/April No 126.

Curran, C. and Grimshaw, C. (2004) Guide to the Mental Capacity Bill 2003. *Openmind*, July.

Curran, C. Grimshaw, C. and Hewitt, C. (1999) The Nearest Relative Under the 1983 Mental Health Act. *Openmind* May/June, No 97, p.24.

Curran, C., Grimshaw, C. and Hewitt, D. (1999) The 1983 Mental Health Act Revised Code of Practice: Some implications for Approved Social Workers. *Community Care* 8 July, pp. 28–9.

Curran, C., Grimshaw, C. and Hewitt, D. (2001) The Human Rights Act and mental health law. *Openmind*, May/June, No 109, pp.24–5.

Curran, C., Grimshaw, C. and Zigmond, A. (1997) The doctor's holding power under section 5(2) *Openmind* No 83, p.28.

Curran, C. and Hewitt, D. (2002) National Care Standards Commission and independent psychiatric hospitals. *Openmind*, March/April, No 114, pp. 28–9.

Dein , S. (1997), Clinical review. ABC of mental health: mental health in a multiethnic society, *British Medical Journal*.

Department of Health (1990) *National Health Service and Community Care Act*. London: DoH.

Department of Health (1993) *The Health of the Nation: A strategy for health in England*. London: HMSO.

Department of Health (1995) *Building Bridges Report*. London: DoH.

Department of Health (1995) *A Handbook on Child and Adolescent Mental Health*. London: HMSO.

Department of Health (1998) *Modernising Mental Health Services: National Priorities Guidance 1999/00–2001/02* LAC(98)22.

Department of Health (1998) *Modernising Mental Health Services: Safe, sound and supportive*. London: DoH.

Department of Health (1998) *Partnerships in Action: New opportunities for joint working between health and social services: a discussion document*. London: DoH.

Department of Health (1999) *Code of Practice to the Mental Health Act 1983 (revised 1999)*. Norwich: Stationery Office.

Department of Health (1999) *National Service Framework for Mental Health – Modern Standards and Service Models*. London: DoH.

Department of Health (1999) *Quality Protects Programme: Transforming children's services 2000–01* LAC (99) 33, London: HMSO.

Department of Health (1999) *The Mental Health Act 1983 Revised Code of Practice*, London: DoH.

Department of Health (1999) *Safer Services: National confidential inquiry into suicide and homicide by people with mental illness*. London: DoH.

Department of Health (2000) *The NHS Plan: a plan for investment: a plan for reform.* London:HMSO.

Department of Health (2001) *Safeguarding Children in Whom Illness is Induced or Fabricated by Carers with Parenting Responsibilities*. London: HMSO.

Department of Health (2001) *Treatment Choice in Psychological Therapies and Counselling: Evidence based clinical practice guidelines*. London: DoH.

Department of Health (2001) *Valuing People: A new strategy for learning disability for the 21st century*. London: TSO.

Department of Health (2002) *A Sign of the Times: Modernising mental health services for people who are deaf*. London: DoH.

Department of Health (2002) *Dual Diagnosis Good Practice Guide*. London: TSO.

Department of Health (2002) *Mental Health Implementation Guide: Dual diagnosis good practice guide*. London: DoH.

Department of Health (2001) *The Mental Health Policy Implementation Guide*. London: DoH.

Department of Health (2003) *Delivering Race Equality: A framework for Action*. Consultation Document. London: DoH.

Department of Health (1999) *Effective Care Co-Ordination in Mental Health Services: Modernising the Care Programme Approach – a policy booklet*. London: DoH.

Department of Health (2003) *Skills for Health*. London: DoH.

Department of Health (2003) *Women's Mental Health: Into the mainstream: strategic development of mental health care for women*. London: DoH.

Department of Health (2004) *An Easy Guide to Direct Payments*. London: TSO.

Department of Health, (2006), White Paper – Our health, our care, our say: A new direction for community services. 30 January.

Department of Health (2004) Core Document, National Service Framework for Children, Young People and Maternity Services.

Dogra, N., Parkin, A., Gale, F. and Frake, C.(2001) *A Multidisciplinary Handbook of Child and Adolescent Mental Health for Front Line Professionals*. London: Jessica Kingsley.

Dominelli, L, (1988) *Anti–Racist Social Work. A challenge for white practitioners and educators*. Basingstoke: Macmillan.

Double D, (2006) *Critical Psychiarty: Limits of Madness*, New York. Palgrave Macmillan.

European Commission (2005) Green Paper – Improving the mental health of the population: Towards a strategy on mental health for the European Union.

Eldergill, A. (1997) *Mental Health Law Review Tribunals: Law and practice*. Sweet and Maxwell: London.

Epstein, S. (1983) Natural healing processes of the mind, in J. Newton (1988), *Preventing Mental Illness*, London: Routledge.

Fernado, S. Ethnicity and Mental Health in M. Ulas, and A. Connor (1999) *Mental Health and Social Work*. London: Jessica Kinglsey.

Findings (2004) Understanding What Children Say About Living with Domestic Violence, Parental Substance Misuse or Parental Health Problems. York: JRF.

Finzen, A. (2002) in S. Priebe, and M. Slade *Evidence in Mental Health Care*. Hove: Brunner-Routledge.

Fox, C. and Hawton, K. (2004) *Deliberate Self-Harm in Adolescence*. London: Jessica Kingsley.

Frangou, S. and Bryne, P. (2000) How to manage the first episode of schizophrenia. *British Medical Journal* 321 (7260):522.

Fulford, K.W.M. (2004a), Ten principles of values-based practice (VBP), in Radden (ed.) *Companion to the Philosophy of Psychiatry*. New York: Oxford University Press.

Fulford, K.W.M. (2004b) Values in Mental Health Services, in Mental Health Act Commission Tenth Biennial Report 2001–3. Norwich: Stationery Office.

Gilbert ,P. (2003), *The Value of Everything: Social work and its importance in the field of mental health*. Lyme Regis: Russell House Publishing.

Glover, K. in T. Bassett and S. Cuthbert (2000) *Certificate in Community Mental Health*. Student's workbook. Southampton: Ashford Press.

Goffman, E. (1961) *Asylums*. London: Penguin.

Golightley, T.M. (1985) *If Only They Would Listen: The case for a community orientated mental health service*. Lincoln: University of Lincoln.

Gomm, R. (2004) *Social Research Methodology: critical introduction*. Basingstoke: Palgrave Macmillan.

Gottlieb, B. (ed) (1981) *Social Networks and Social Support*. London: Sage.

Griffiths, R. (1988) *Community Care: Agenda for Action*. London: HMSO.

GSCC (2002) *Codes of Practice for Social Care Workers and Employers*. London: General Social Care Council.

Health Advisory Service (1994) *Suicide Prevention: The challenge confronted*. London: HMSO.

Health Advisory Service (1995) *Child and Adolescent Mental Health Services – Together We Stand*. London: HMSO.

Health Advisory Service (2001) *Substance Misuse and Mental Health Comorbity (Dual Diagnosis): Standards for Mental Health Services*. London: HAS.

Hewitt, D. (2005) An inconvenient mirror – do we already have the next Mental Health Act. *Journal of Mental Health Law* November pp. 138–49.

Horner, N. (2003) *What is Social Work? Context and perspectives*. Exeter: Learning Matters.

Huxley, P. (1985) *Social Work Practice in Mental Health*. Aldershot: Gower.

Huxley, P. (2002) Evidence in social care, in S. Priebe and M. Slade, *Evidence in Mental Health Care*. Hove: Brunner-Routledge.

James, J. (2003) *Seeing Through Walls: A report on social inclusion in practice based on the findings of the Social Inclusion Mapping Exercise*. Durham: Northern Centre for Mental Health.

Johns, R. (2003) *Using the Law in Social Work*. Exeter; Learning Matters.

Jones, K. (1993) *Asylums and After: A revised history of the mental health services from the early 18th century to the 1900s*. London: Athlone Press.

Jones, K. et al. (1985) *After Hospital: A study of long term psychiatric patients in York*. York: York District Health Authority.

Jones, R. (2002) *Mental Health Act Manual* (8th ed). London: Sweet and Maxwell.

Joseph Rowntree Foundation (2004) *Mental Health Service Users and their Involvement in Risk Assessment and Management*. York: JRF ref. 414.

Kalfi, Y. and Torabi, M. (1996) The Role of Parental 'Expressed Emotion' in Relapse of Schizophrenia. *Iran Journal of Medicine*: 21(1 72): 46.

Keating, F. and Robertson, D. (2002) Breaking the circles of fear: a review of mental health services to African and Caribbean communities, in *Your Shout: Mental Health Promotion*, Issue 4. pp. 18–19.

Kim, W.J. (1995) A training guideline of cultural competence for child and adolescent psychiatric residencies. *Child Psychiatry and Human Development* 26:2, 125–36.

Kreitman, N. (1997) *Parasuicide*. Chichester: Wiley.

Laing, R.D. (1985) *Wisdom, madness and folly. The making of a psychiatrist*. Basingstoke: Macmillan.

Langan, J. and Lindow, V. (2004) *Living with Risk: Mental health service user involvement in risk assessment and management*. Bristol: Policy Press.

Leff, J., Kuipers, K. and Lam, D. (2002) *Family Work for Schizophrenia* (2nd ed). London: Royal College of Psychiatrists.

Low, J. (2004) *Lay acquiescence to medical dominance in assessing the efficacy of alternative and complementary therapies: reflections on the active citizenship thesis*. Paper presented to the European Sociological Association Symposium on Professions, Social Inclusion and Citizenship. Lincoln: University of Lincoln.

MacLean, M. (2004) *Together and Apart: Children and parents experiencing divorce*. York: JRF (Foundations series).

Mckeown, M. and Mercer, D. (1998) Language, race and forensic psychiatry, in T. Mason, and C. Mercer, (eds) *Critical Perspectives in Forensic Care*. Basingstoke: Macmillan.

Menninger, K. (1963) *The Vital Balance: The life process in mental health and illness*. London: Viking Press.

Mental Health Act Commission (1999–2001) *Ninth Biennial Report*. London: Stationery Office.

Mental Health Foundation (1999) *The Big Picture: Promoting children and young people's mental health*. London: Mental Health Foundation.

Mischon, J. (2000) Report of the independent inquiry team into the care and treatment of Daniel Joseph. Sutton and Wandsworth Health Authority and Lambeth, Southwark and Lewisham Health Authority.

Modestein and Schwarzenbach (1992) Effect of psycho–pharmacotherapy on suicide risk in discharged psychiatric patients, Acta Psychiatrica Scandinavia in C. Pritchard (1995) *Suicide – The Ultimate Rejection*. Buckingham: Open University Press.

Nazroo, J. (1999) *Ethnicity and Mental Health*. London: Policy Studies Institute.

Neustatter, A. (2003) Changing shapes, in *Young Minds Magazine*, No 68 .

Newman, T. and Blackburn, S. (2002) *Transitions in the Lives of Children and Young People: Resilience factors*. Barnardo's Policy, Research and Influencing Unit: Scottish Executive Education Department.

Newton, J. (1988) *Preventing Mental Illness*. London: Routledge.

NIMHE, (2003) Inside outside: improving mental health services for black and minority ethnic communities in England. www.nimhe.org.uk

NIMHE, (2006) National Suicide Prevention Strategy for England: Annual Report on Progress 2005, Care Service Improvement Partnership, Leeds.

O'Hagan, K. (ed) (1996) *Competence in Social Work Practice*. London: Jessica Kingsley.

O'Sullivan, T. (1999) *Decision Making in Social Work*. Basingstoke: Macmillan.

Obafunwa, J.O. and Busuttil, A. (1994) Clinical contact preceding suicide, in C. Pritchard (1995) *Suicide – The Ultimate Rejection*. Buckingham: Open University Press.

Oliver, M. (1996) *Understanding Disability: from theory to practice*. Basingstoke: Macmillan.

Onyett, S. (1992) *Case Management in Mental Health*. Cheltenham: Stanley Thornes.

Orbach, S. (1986) *Hunger Strike*. London: Penguin.

Our Health, our care, our say: A new direction for community services. White Paper accessible at www.dh.gov.uk/ourhealthourcareoursay

Parker, J. and Bradley, G. (2003) *Social Work Practice: Assessment, planning, intervention and review*. Exeter: Learning Matters.

Patel, K. et al. (2003) *Engaging and Changing: Developing effective policy for the care and treatment of black and minority ethnic detained patients*. London: DoH.

Pearce, J. (1999) Collaboration between the NHS and Social Services in the provision of child and adolescent mental health services: a personal view. *Child Psychology and Psychiatry Review*, 4;4, 150–3.

Pharoah F. M., Mari, J. J. and Steiner, D. (2000) *American Journal of Psychiatry*, 153, 607–17 in the Cochrane Library issue 3, 2002, Oxford update software.

Pilgrim, D. and Rogers, A. (1999) *A Sociology of Mental Health and Illness* (2nd ed). Buckingham: Open University Press.

Pollack, W. (1999) *Real Boys*. New York: Henry Holt.

Poole, D.L. (1998) Politically correct or culturally competent, *Health and Social Work*, 23 (3) 163–6.

Priebe, S. and Slade, M. (2002) *Evidence in Mental Health Care*. Hove: Brunner-Routledge.

Prins, H. (1999) *Will They Do It Again?: Risk assessment and management in criminal justice and psychiatry*. London: Routledge.

Pritchard, C. (1995) *Suicide – The Ultimate Rejection*. Buckingham: Open University Press.

Ramon, S. (2001) Opinions and dilemmas facing British mental health social work, in J. Tew, Going social: championing a holistic model of mental distress within professional education, *Social Work Education*, Vol 21 No 2, 2002.

Red Manual Code of Practice (2004) *Section D:10 working with parents with mental health problems*. Lincoln: Lincolnshire County Council.

Rethink, Sane and Zito Trust (2003) Behind Closed Doors: The current state and future of acute mental health care in the UK. London: *Rethink*. www.rethink.org/research/Behind-Closed/Doors.htm

Ridgeway, S.M. (1997) Deaf people and psychological health – some preliminary findings. *Deaf Worlds*, Issue 1, Vol 13, 9–17.

Rikken, M. (1995) A preventive mental health programme for children of parents with mental disorders, in D. Trent, and A. Reed (1995) *Promotion of Mental Health*. Aldershot: Ashgate.

Ritchie, J.H., Dick D. and Lingham, R. (1994) *The Report of the Inquiry into the Care and Treatment of Christopher Clunis*. London: HMSO.

Robbins, D. (2004) *Treated as People: An overview of mental health services from a social care perspective*. London: SSI/DoH.

Rodgers, B. and Pryor, J. (1998) *Divorce and Separation: The outcome for children*. York: JRF.

Rowland, N. and Gross, S. (2003) *Evidence-Based Counselling and Psychological Therapies*. Hove: Brunner-Routledge.

Rutter, M. (1999) *Bright Futures: Promoting children and young people's mental health*. London: Mental Health Foundation.

Sainsbury Centre for Mental Health (1998) *Keys to Engagement: review of care for people with severe mental illness who are hard to engage with services*. London: Sainsbury Centre.

Sainsbury Centre for Mental Health (2002) *Breaking the Circles of Fear*. London: Sainsbury Centre.

Sainsbury Centre for Mental Health (2003) *Mental Health Topics: Assertive outreach*. London: Sainsbury Centre.

Sartorius, N. et al. (1990) *Sources and Traditions of Classification in Psychiatry*. World Health Organisation/Hogrefe and Huber. Toronto: Lewiston.

Schram, A. et al. (1999) *Positive Practice in Mental Health* (2nd ed). Crook: Breakthrough.

Scull, A.T. (1979) *Museums of Madness: The social organisation of insanity in 19th century England*. London: Allen Lane.

Spender, Q. et al. (2001) *Child Mental Health in Primary Care*. Abingdon: Radcliffe Medical Press.

Swinton J (2001) *Spirituality and Mental Health Care*. London: Jessica Kingsley

Szasz, T.S. (1972) *The myth of mental illness*. London: Paladin.

Tew, J. (2002) Going social: championing a holistic model of mental distress within professional education. *Social Work Education*, Vol. 21, no. 2.

Trent D. and Reed, C. (eds) (1995) *Promotion of Mental Health Vol. 4* Aldershot: Avebury.

Trent NHS Strategic Health Authority. (2005) Principles for Practice. December. Available by email request from Rachel.Hawley@tsha.nhs.uk

Tribe, R. and Raval, H. (eds) (2003) *Working with Interpreters in Mental Health*. Hove: Brunner-Routledge.

Ulas, M. and Connor, A. (1999) *Mental Health and Social Work Research Highlights in Social Work 28*. London: Jessica Kingsley .

Walker, S. (2003) *Social Work and Child and Adolescent Mental Health*. Lyme Regis: Russell House Publishing.

Walker, S. (2003) Social work and child mental health: psychological principles in community practice. *British Journal of Social Work* 33: 673–87.

Walker, S. (2003) *Working Together for Healthy Young Minds*. Lyme Regis: Russell House Publishing.

Webb, S. (2006) *Social Work in a Risk Society.* New York: Palgrave Macmillan.

Webster, R. (1996) *Why Freud Was Wrong: Science, sin and psychoanalysis*, London: HarperCollins.

Weal, A. (1999) *Adolescence: Positive approaches for working with young people*. Lyme Regis: Russell House Publishing.

WHO (2001) World Health Report, p11.http://www.who.int/whr/2001

Williams, R. and Morgan, G. (eds) (1994) *Suicide Prevention: The challenge confronted*. London: HMSO.

Yelloly, M.A. (1980) *Social Work Theory and Psychoanalysis*. Wokingham: Van Nostrand Rheinhold.

Index

A

A Sign of the Times: Modernising mental health services (DoH) 13
active phase, schizophrenia 28
adolescents
    compulsory admissions 81–2
    engaging and communicating with 83
    mental disorders
        common 76–8
        nature and extent of 76–8
    mental health 74–5
    social exclusion 82
    social work
        interventions 79–80
        knowledge needed 72–3
        services 80–1
advance directives 53–4
Afro-Caribbean people
    compulsory detention of 12
    diagnosis of schizophrenia 28
    over-representation in secondary care 10
alcohol misuse 31–2
Allitt Inquiry 140–1
alternative therapies 27, 90
Alzheimer's disease 32
    features associated with 32
    social work role 33
    treatment and management 32
anorexia nervosa 79, 86
anti-depressants 27, 30–1, 109
anti-oppressive practice 12–14
anti-psychotics 27
Anti-Racist Social Work 12
appeals, against detention 61
applicants, compulsory admission 50–1
applications
    compulsory admission 52–3
    guardianship 64
approved doctor 153, 156
approved social workers 46, 153
    admissions to hospital 48–9

duties and powers 48
    warrant to search 55
Assertive Outreach 125, 130
assessments 24
    attempted suicide 101–3
    compulsory admissions 51
    long-term users with schizophrenia 116–22
    see also Child Assessment Orders; Community Care Assessment; psychiatric assessment tools; risk assessment
attempted suicide, working with 101–4
attention deficit hyperactivity disorder 77
autonomy 9

B

Beck Depression Inventory 25
behaviour modification 77, 153
behavioural signs, eating disorders 88–9
best interests, compulsory admission 53
bipolar affective disorder 31, 76
black service users, discrimination 10–12
body shape, eating disorders 86
Bolam test 153
boxes technique 19
British National Formulary 153
British Sign Language 13
bulimia 84

C

Camberwell Family Interview (CFI) 128–9
CAMHS handbook 81
capacity *see* mental capacity
care *see* community care; mental health care; primary care
care orders 141
care plans 130
Care Programme Approach (CPA) 62–3, 123, 124
carers, caring for 130

Carers (Recognition and Services Act)
(1995) 104
Caribbean people see Afro-Caribbean
people
Child Assessment Orders 141
child mental health teams 138
child protection 141–50
children
assessment of risk and resilience 148–9
compulsory admissions 81–2
mental disorders
common 76–8
effects of parents' 146
nature and extent of 74–5
safeguarding from fabricated or
induced 147
mental health, parental separation 143–4
social exclusion 82
social work
interventions 79–80
knowledge needed 72–3
services 80–1
understanding 147–8
Children Act (1989) 135, 141
Chlorpromazine 27
citizen participation 135
civil liberty, compulsory detention 60–1
classification, mental disorders 25–6
'clinical iceberg' 35
Cochrane Centre 37
Code of Practice (MHA) 7, 12, 45, 51, 53,
60, 61, 81
cognitive behaviour therapy 76, 90, 108,
153
Commission for Health, Audit and
Inspection (2004) 153
Commission for Social Care and Inspection
4, 153
community
reintegration in 125
treatment in 62–4
community based teams 63
community care 104–5, 118–20
Community Care Assessment 105
Community Care (Direct Payments) Act
(1996) 105, 106
Community Mental Health Trusts 63
community psychiatric nurses 154

complaints procedure 110
compulsory admission
children and adolescents 81–2
criteria 52–3
framework for 45–8
medical recommendations 49–52
through the courts 55–7
Conexions 144
Confidential Inquiry into Homicides and
Suicides by Mentally Ill People 97
confidentiality 9
consent 58
counselling 77
Court of Protection 62, 153
courts, compulsory admission through 55–6
CPA see Care Programme Approach
crisis services 107, 108
cultural competence 2, 14, 15–18

D
dangerousness 118–20
deaf people 13–14
decision making 66–7
Delivering Race Equality: A Framework for
Action 11
delusions 28, 121–2
depression 30
bipolar affective disorder 31, 76
children and adolescents 76
features associated with 30
in mothers after childbirth 144
in older people 32
social work role 29
and suicide 98–104
treatment and management 29
detention, in hospital 57–9, 60–1
diagnosis 25, 154
Diagnostic and Statistical Manual of Mental
Disorders see DSM–IV
diet, and eating disorders 84
difference, understanding 17
Direct Payments scheme 105, 106
Director of Social Services 46
Disability Discrimination Act (1995) 19
Disability Discrimination Act (1999) 13
discharge
from hospital 60–2
supervised 64–5

discrimination 10–11, 17
disease model *see* medical model
dissociative disorders 78, 92
Dissociative Experiences Scale (DES) 78
diversity 8, 17
drift theory 35
drug misuse 31
drugs, costs of 58
DSM-IV 25, 76
dual diagnosis 31–2, 123

E
eating disorders 79, 84
    early warning signs 89
    factors lying behind 85–6
    interventions 88–9
    social work response 86
    websites 92–3
electroconvulsive therapy (ECT) 26, 59
emergency treatment 59
emotional signs, eating disorders 88
empowerment 8, 109, 149
enhanced CPA 62
essential powers 64
ethical dilemmas 9
ethnicity 10–11
Every Child Matters 134, 142
evidence-based practice 36, 150
expressed emotion 128, 154

F
family therapy 128, 154
financial affairs, management of 62

G
General Social Care Council 7, 46
guardianship 64–5

H
H v Mental Health Review Tribunal 61
hallucinations 28
health and safety, compulsory admission 47
hearing voices, working with people who
    are 121–2
Home Office Mental Health Unit 56, 154
hospital managers 154
Hospital Manager's Review 60–1, 154–5

hospitals
    admissions *see* compulsory admission
    alternatives services 107–8
    detention in 57–9
    leaving 60–2
    see also Medium Secure Hospitals
human rights, admission process 56–7
Human Rights Act (1998) 11, 109
hyperkinetic disorders 77

I
ICD-10 25–6, 31
inpatient interventions 90
inclusive approach 2
individual freedom, *v* public safety 45
individual need 111–12
informal patients 57, 122
information, for detained patients 57
inner cities, incidence of schizophrenia 35
inquiries, learning from 139–41
inspection standards 3
integrated services 37, 137–8
interagency collaboration 123–4, 137
interim care orders 141
International Classification of Diseases
        Volume 10 *see* ICD-10
interventions *see* social work; treatment

K
knowledge, social work practice 3–4

L
labelling theory 35
ladder of participation 135–6
learning disability 22
legislation, need for 44–5
Lettieri scale 100
lithium 31
long-term service users, with schizophrenia
        115–32
    Assertive Outreach 130
    assessment 117–20
    care plans 130–1
    caring for carers 130
    hospital visits 120
    hospitalisation 122–3
    initial contact 116

interventions
early 126
family-based 128–9
interagency working 123–4
trigger events 126–7
understanding impact of 120–1

M
manic depression 31, 76
media messages 11, 23, 118
medical model 22, 24
medical practice 8
medical recommendations 49–50
medication 27
attention deficit hyperactivity disorder 77
depression 30, 76
in hospitals 58–9
right to stop taking 9
schizophrenia 28–9, 126–7
Medium Secure Hospitals, ethnic
detainees 10
mental capacity
compulsory admission 52–3
Mental Capacity Act 2005 67–8
mental disorders
children and adolescents
common 76–8
nature and extent of 74–5
safeguarding from fabricated or
induced 147
defined 22
effect of parents 146
media coverage 11, 23, 118
medical model 22, 24
nature or degree of 49
psycho-social model 35–7
social model 23, 34–5
understanding major forms of 28–34
mental health
adolescent development 73–5
deaf people 13–14
defined 22
effective support systems 41–2
and ethnicity 10–11
explaining 23
National Service Framework 3, 11, 123–4
promoting personal 18–19

promoting positive 39–40
promoting well-being 39
Mental Health Act (1983) 9, 45, 46, 55–6,
57, 58, 62, 141–3, 154
Mental Health Act Commission 10, 46, 81,
154
Mental Health Bill 44, 66
Mental Health Programme Approach (CPA)
62–3
mental health interpreters 52
Mental Health (Patients in the Community)
Act (1995) 45, 64
mental health professionals, management
of 138
Mental Health Review Tribunals 12, 56, 61,
64, 155
Mental Health Services
alternatives to hospital 107
children and adolescents 80–1
interagency collaboration 123–4
learning from inquiries 137–9
service user involvement 135–6
mental illness see mental disorders
MIND 135
Modernisation Plan 11
Modernising Mental Health Services
(DoH) 3
mood disorders see depression
mothers, risk of depression 144
multidisciplinary teams 137
multiple personality disorder 78
Munchausen's Syndrome by Proxy 140
Museums of Madness 22

N
National Care Standards Commission
(NCSC) 153
National Health Service and Community
Care Act (1990) 6, 104, 110, 135
National Institute for Clinical Excellence
(NICE) 59, 155
National Institute for Mental Health
Excellence (NIMHE) 16, 97, 155
National Occupational Standards 1
National Service Framework 3, 11, 124
National Workforce Action Team 138
nearest relatives 51, 155
NHS Plan 3

normative principles 6

O

old age, depression 32, 98–107
onset schizophrenia 29
organic disorders 32
Our Healthier Nation 39

P

parental separation, children's mental
    health 143
Parenting Matters 140
parents
    effect of mental disorders on
      children 146
    psycho-social educational approach
      with parents 149
paternalism 9
patient advocacy services 10
Percy Commission (1957) 48
personal factors 149
phenomenological approach 25
Police and Criminal Evidence Act (1984) 54
police powers 54
political approach, promoting mental
    health 39
poverty, mental disorder 35
pre-adolescent children, mental health
    problems 73
pre-onset schizophrenia 29
predisposing factors 36, 38
Present State Examination (PSE) 25
primary care 81
primary deviance 35
prisons, drug use 31
prodromal phase, schizophrenia 29
protection of others, compulsory admission
    49–50
Prozac 30
psychiatric assessment tools 23, 103
psychiatric hospitals see hospitals
psychiatric morbidity survey (ONS) 22
psychiatrists 25
psychoanalysis 155
psychological debriefing 37
psychological factors 36, 37, 148
psychological therapies 26
    see also behaviour modification;

cognitive behaviour therapy;
    counselling; family therapy;
    psychotherapy
psycho-social context, social work 37–40
psycho-social interventions 37, 90, 108,
    149
psycho-social model 34, 149
psychosurgery 26
psychotherapy 77, 90
Public Guardianship Office 62, 155
public places 54
public safety, v individual freedom 45

R

R on the application of Colonel Munjaz v
    Mersey Care NHS Trust 59
Race Relations (Amendment) Act (2000) 11
relapse, schizophrenia 128
research reports 150
residual phase, schizophrenia 29
resilience 148–9
responsible local social services
    authority 64
responsible medical officers 60, 155
restraint 59
restriction orders 56
'revolving door' admissions 52
right to refuse treatment 9–10, 58, 122
risk, media messages 23
risk assessment
    child protection 141–8
    involving service users 120
    suicide 100–4
Ritalin 77
Royal National Institute for Deaf People 13

S

S v Airedale NHS Trust (2003) 59
Sainsbury Centre 130
schizophrenia 28
    costs of treatment 58
    features associated with 29
    long term users 116–31
    prognosis 29
    social causation 34–5
    social work role 29
    symptoms 28
    treatment and management 29

school age children, mental health
    problems 73, 145
seclusion 59
second opinion appointed doctor 156
secondary deviance 32
Section 12 approved doctor 156
self-awareness 14
self-disclosure, limited 8
self-harm 78
self-help 78, 106
service users
    empowerment 8, 109, 149
    involvement of 135–6
    see also black service users; deaf people;
        long-term service users; short-term
        service users
short-term powers 54
short-term service users 95–113
    alternative to hospital based services
        107–8
    depression and suicide 98–107
    interventions 108–110
    monitoring and reviewing plans 112
    policy context 96–7
    providing for individual need 111–12
skills 4, 17
social causation factors 34–5, 36, 38,
        99–100, 148
Social Circumstances Reports 12
social exclusion 3, 13, 82–3
social model 23, 35–6
social work
    Alzheimer's disease 32
    anti-oppressive practice 12
    with children and adolescents
        interventions 79–80
        knowledge needed 72–3
    cultural competence 15–18
    depression 30–1
    dual diagnosis 31–2
    eating disorders 84–5
    psycho-social context 37–40
    schizophrenia 29
    suicide 98–9
social work reports 61
social workers
    CPA 62–4
    see also approved social workers
Special Educational Needs and Disability
        Act (2001) 19

standard CPA 62
standards, NSF 3–4, 124
statutory duty 156
statutory instrument 156
stereotypical views 16
stimulant medication 77
stress
    as intervening variable 38
    managing while studying 91
    personal mental health 18–19
    preventing 39–40
structural racism 17
Structured Clinical Interview (SCID–D) 78
student mental health 18–19
substance misuse 31, 123
suicide
    and depression 98–104
    national targets
        Confidential Inquiry 97
        reduction 39, 97
        workforce 97–8
    statistics 96–7
supervised discharge 64
support systems
    preventing stress 41–2
    short-term service users 106
Supporting Families 142
Sure Start projects 145
system failure 119
systematic reviews 37

T
test of capacity 67
Thorn Initiative 128
thought insertion 28
Together and Apart 143
treatment 26–7
    advance refusal of 53–4
    Alzheimer's disease 32
    in the community 62–4
    depression 30–1, 108–10
    eating disorders 90
    in hospital 58–60
    right to refuse 58, 122
    schizophrenia 28
    see also medication
trigger events 126–7

U
under-5s, problems associated with 73
Using the Law in Social Work (2003) 141

V
values
  in action 8
  importance of 6–7
Valuing People 6
Victoria Climbié case 139–40

violence, media messages 23
voices, hearing 121–2

W
warrant to search 55
workforce programme 97–8, 138

Y
YoungMinds 135, 145